Transplanted

Surviving
Type 1 Diabetes
and Kidney Failure

Janice S. Zunde

Transplanted

Surviving Type 1 Diabetes and Kidney Failure

For more information, contact Janice S. Zunde at janzundehealth@gmail.com
The content of this book is majorly for general instruction only. Each person's physical, emotional and spiritual condition is unique. The information in this book is not intended to replace or interrupt the reader's relationship with a physician or other professional. Please consult your doctor for matters pertaining to your specific health and diet.

Or visit www.janicezundehealth.com

ISBN-13: 978-1530125609 (CreateSpace-Assigned)
ISBN-10: 153012560X
Library of Congress Control Number:LCCN: 2016904584

Printed by CreateSpace Publishing
CreateSpace Independent Publishing Platform,
North Charleston, SC
Printed and Bound in the United States of America

Dedication

This book is dedicated to
my beloved people in the world, my husband Steve and
my daughter Gaby.

You are both my inspiration and motivation
in everything I do.

"I learned that courage was not the absence of fear, but the triumph over it. I felt fear myself more times than I can remember, but I hid behind a mask of boldness. The brave man is not he who does not feel afraid, but he who conquers that fear."

Mandela, Nelson Oct,1995: *Long Walk to Freedom*

Contents

Introduction

At seven years old, I was diagnosed with type 1 diabetes. I had been losing weight, drinking gallons of water and feeling exhausted constantly for several weeks on end.

We had celebrated Guy Fawkes Day a few months prior. Guy Fawkes is a traditional holiday in South Africa (also called Bonfire Night and Fireworks Night) observed on the fifth of November every year. It involves a lot of firecrackers and fireworks. My brother's friend threw a Guy Fawkes Day firecracker at me during the festivities. The firecracker exploded near my face. Fortunately, I was not hurt, but it is commonly believed that type 1 diabetes is precipitated by a physical trauma. It is impossible to know if this is what triggered it, because there was no genetic predisposition for diabetes in my family.

It has been found that "50 percent of autoimmune disorders have been attributed to unknown trigger factors. Physical and psychological stress has been implicated in the development of autoimmune diseases. Not only that, but the treatment of autoimmune diseases should include stress management and behavioral intervention."[1]

We had recently returned from our annual vacation to Durban in Natal Province, South Africa, and I had been feeling particularly tired. I laid down on my bed and slipped into a diabetic coma. Fortunately, Uncle Bertie, our family friend as well as our primary care physician, realized the gravity of my situation and rushed me off to the children's hospital in Johannesburg. I remained there for a month to acclimate and adjust to my new situation.

The Mayo Clinic defines type 1 diabetes, which is also known as juvenile diabetes, as "a chronic condition in which the pancreas produces little or no insulin, a hormone needed to allow sugar to enter the body cells in order to facilitate the production of energy."[2]

The glucose continuously circulates in the blood and leaves one feeling lethargic, sleepy, and with extreme brain fog. Because the glucose can't get into the body cells and builds up in the bloodstream, it puts the body into crisis. The most common symptoms of undiagnosed type 1 diabetes are significant weight loss, extreme fatigue and irritability, constant urination, thirst and blurred vision.

At first, I was in complete denial and was determined to carry on with life despite my diagnosis. These were

---

1   Stojanovi L, , Marisavljevich D Stress as a Trigger for Autoimmunity, January 2008 University Medical Center, Belgrade University, Serbia

2   Mayo clinic staff, , diabetes-symptoms, http://www.mayoclinic.org/diseases-conditions/diabetes/in-depth/June 2013

the days before blood glucose monitoring and insulin pumps. At the time, a urine test was the only way to gauge my blood sugar. We now know this is a primitive and entirely inaccurate means of assessing blood sugar, and no one would dream of using this today as a means of assessment.

Diet became an ongoing issue for me. My endocrinologist put me on a very restricted diet, as well as insulin shots.

In a conversation with my mother as an adult, she told me, "The first time I had to give you an injection, I gave it to you and then ran to the bathroom and was immediately sick." We used the old-fashioned types of glass syringes that needed to be decontaminated every time after use. Not the quick disposable ones used today. I have a distinct memory of a large silver sterilizer, placed in one corner of our kitchen, plugged into an outlet in the wall, bubbling with steaming water, where my mother would put the used syringes.

My mother brought me lunch every day to school to ensure that I was eating regularly, in accordance with the diet the doctor had recommended. Sandwiches made on thick slices of whole-wheat bread, with generous portions of cold cuts were (unbeknownst to my mother) switched out for much more exciting sandwiches of marshmallow fluff and sprinkles, made on fluffy white bread.

Her goal was to ensure that I was eating plenty of protein (probably way too much according to today's standards) to counteract smaller amounts of carbohydrate. I also ate plenty of vegetables and limited fruits.

I would always sneak into the "forbidden" candy and cakes in an act of rebellion. This created havoc on my blood sugar levels, but didn't stop me from enjoying the treats that all of my friends were eating.

Being a caring mom, my mother was just following the doctor's orders. I was too young to fully comprehend and appreciate the efforts my mother made to take care of me. I had no idea she was scared too.

The emotional aspect of taking care of a type 1 diabetic child was sadly not a consideration in those days. Neither was the new family dynamic and the effect on my siblings, who seemed confused and somewhat envious of all the attention I received.

My brother, sister and I would arrive home from a long day at school and sit for a lunch prepared by my mother or Dora, our beloved housekeeper. Lunch at home consisted of a full meal. Spaghetti Bolognese, fried fish and chips, baby lamb chops and chips, monkey gland steak (nothing at all to do with monkey gland, but a traditional fragrant and slightly spicy South African sauce, served with steak), or chicken a la king were a few of the commonly lunches we enjoyed. All were served with a colorful, bountiful salad.

After a long day at school, these sumptuous meals were welcomed and enjoyed, and they piqued my interest in cooking. The kitchen has always been a place of intrigue for me. It was where the magic happened. My mother spent hours in the kitchen, following recipes, and often creating her own. Friends happily and eagerly followed us home from school to join us for lunch and often stayed on for dinner.

This is how my journey began, as well as my struggle to achieve health and vitality, despite the challenges that faced me. Every stage of my life came with new challenges. Balancing all life's ups and downs is difficult at the best of times, but having diabetes makes it more difficult.

My journey through pregnancy, kidney/pancreas transplant, renal failure, dialysis, and finally to radiant health and vitality has been interwoven with diet and nutrition. Throughout the different stages of my life, I had to periodically adapt my diet to stay on top of my health, and I later began to realize that there was a new paradigm in play.

Once I started studying integrative nutrition through the Institute of Integrative Nutrition® in 2014, it finally all made sense to me. I began to understand how to keep healthy, despite all I had been through medically. My interest in organic, real, clean food intensified, and along with that, my love of experimenting with new, more updated ways of cooking developed and expanded.

I also began to understand that the food we eat is only secondary to how we take care of ourselves mentally and physically. By undertaking self-care in the form of meditation, yoga, massage, and our relationships with our loved ones, we take care of ourselves on a much deeper level. This is our primary source of food. It is what lifts us up, energizes and nourishes us, besides the food on our plates.

I knew it was crucial to follow my doctor's orders and to continue taking my medications regularly as prescribed. But it was equally important to eat organic, real food uncontaminated by pesticides and herbicides, not genetically modified or factory farmed, processed and administered growth hormones.

As Michael Pollan, American author, journalist, activist and professor of journalism at the UC Berkeley Graduate School of Journalism said, "If it came from a plant, eat it; if it was made in a plant, don't." [3]

I am a firm believer that whatever happens to us in life is a learning experience to foster personal growth. It is essential not to feel victimized by our experiences, but instead, to take them positively and learn from them.

This book is a celebration of life and survival. I feel motivated and compelled to share what I have experienced and learned in the last 50 years since my initial diagnosis, and hopefully, it will motivate and help others with similar challenges.

Combining a healthy diet with living a balanced, healthy lifestyle is the key to living a long, vibrant and healthy life. This book and the recipes that go along with it are my story.

---

[3]   Pollan, Michael Dec 2009 *Food Rules: An Eaters Manual*

Part 1.

CHAPTER 1.

Living with Childhood Diabetes

Growing up in South Africa in the 60s and 70s, we were privileged to have a housekeeper take care of us, and help my mother with household chores. Dora was a crucial part of my childhood, and I greatly adored her.

Dora took care of all three of us from birth, and was our regular companion from the time we woke up in the morning, until the time we retired to bed at night. She would delight us with marvelous stories, featuring Dom Jan and Slim Jan, the silly brother and the clever brother, at night, while our parents worked at our family-owned cinema.

Dora was an African woman from Rustenburg, a city about three hours away from where we lived. Her two daughters still resided at her home while she worked and lived with us. She was only able to see them a few times a year. Many young African women lived in that manner, sending what they earned as live-in domestic workers to their families every month.

She was our unofficial second mother. She was there when we scraped our knees in the park, and when we came home from school tired and hungry. She was always a constant, comforting and consoling presence in our day-to-day lives, and took care of us as if we were her own children. Occasionally, Dora's husband would visit her. The visits often ended with a drunken beating and consequent police raid. He often landed in prison for several weeks, leaving Dora bruised and battered until the next visit. This was the sad reality for many African women during the Apartheid era. They were set apart from their children and were often victims of substance abuse and violence.

When I was a toddler, Dora carried me on her back, wrapped in a blanket, as was the custom in South Africa. I would fall asleep with my head resting against her shoulder blades. My mother still jokingly blames Dora for my bow-leggedness, accusing her of carrying me strapped around her back for way too long.

There was an extra special bond between Dora and me. She would brush and braid my hair before school every day and then walk me and my siblings to and from our local elementary school, which was about ten minutes away. Dora always accompanied us to the park, and would regale us all afterwards with tales of our antics on the swings.

Unfortunately for us, it was necessary for Dora to return home for good to her children. I cried inconsolably for days. I was completely heartbroken after she left us, and was sure that I would never recover from her absence and my heartache.

Dora's departure just happened to coincide with my diagnosis of type 1 diabetes. The effect of stress on our bodies is an interesting topic. It is a known fact that stress can trigger a myriad of symptoms in one's body, including an autoimmune reaction. I often wonder if this could this have been the trigger for me.

Being a high-profile Jewish family in a small town called Florida, where my father owned a local movie theater, it was not surprising that we encountered many bouts of anti-Semitism. Naturally, the fact that we had access to free movies was a big draw regarding popularity. But I remember waiting for my brother after school one day. After looking for him for hours, I found him at the playground, surrounded by a group of boys who were pushing him around, kicking him and calling him a "bloody Jew."

After elementary school, I went to a Jewish Day School in Johannesburg, called King David Victory Park, where I no longer experienced the anti-Semitism that I had encountered previously. I loved school from this point on, and the difference was enormous. My education in this nurturing environment allowed me to grow and flourish, giving me the confidence and courage to survive the many difficulties that would come my way in the years to come.

Dancing three times a week at our local dance studio, under the stern and watchful eye of Isabelle Maybury, our dancing teacher, was part of my sister Bonita's and my life from the time we were five years old. I was a plump child and was constantly teased and taunted by Isabelle.

My frustration turned to guilt that I was in some way responsible for being overweight. I would sometimes be excluded from participating in certain dances during festivals and competitions because I did not "fit in" with the other girls. Eventually, when I was in high school, I decided to quit dancing, an art form that I loved, due to Isabelle's abusive, ignorant and cruel treatment.

The emphasis on weight, and the assumption that I was responsible for being slightly overweight, was rooted in "sheer ignorance," as Kerri Sparling, type 1 diabetes blogger and author of "Balancing Diabetes," said in an interview with Brian Mowll, MD. The stigma made me unworthy of empathy and value in my dancing teacher's eyes.

I felt isolated in my diagnosis. I did not know any other children with type 1 diabetes and society seemed to perpetuate my struggle of acceptance.

There was no support group to meet others in the same boat, and or an online community in those days. I was utterly alone in making sense of an unfair world. In those days, no one suggested any form of assistance or psycho-education to deal with this emotional heartache. Therapy was a foreign concept in South Africa in 1970.

Today, seeking the help of a professional such as a psychologist, dietitian or a health coach like me, to guide you step by step in managing your diabetes is crucial. It is important to find someone who can feel your frustrations and challenges in managing this unpredictable disease.

I had to work much harder, since I did not have that support, to achieve what everyone else took for granted. All I wanted was to be treated like every other child, and not be given "special" treatment or to be excluded.

During summer vacations, both my older brother and my younger sister went to a sleep-away camp for three weeks. I wished that I could be bundled off along with them, make new friends, and have fun at the beach.

Year after year, the ritual continued of seeing them off at the train station, with me remaining back home, feeling sad and isolated. It felt punitive and exclusive to be denied this privilege, all because I was a diabetic child.

During my final year of high school, I began going to Weight Watchers International and started losing weight, dramatically. My weight dropped from 130 lbs. to approximately 100 lbs. over a period of two years.

No one suspected this dramatic weight loss to be the result of very high blood sugar. Back then we did not have glucometers to monitor fluctuations in blood sugar levels. Keeping control of blood sugar for a type 1 diabetic in 1965 was pretty much like shooting in the dark. A urine stick was the sole means of assessment. It was a completely inferior and inaccurate gauge.

I was encouraged by one and all to "carry on the good work" of losing weight. I became dangerously skinny, but my parents, pediatrician and everyone else appeared to cheer me on. My sister did approach me about this dramatic weight loss, but I became defensive and insisted that I was perfectly fine. I had made a lot of friends at this time, and I excelled academically so superficially everything looked great.

The havoc in my body was unseen and unimaginable, with future damage to my eyes and kidneys to come. The first time that I became aware of the potential danger ahead was when I changed doctors.

My new endocrinologist, Larry Distiller, MD, had just come back from studying in the US and took over my care. He made an all-out effort to change my thinking about diabetic care and management. From two shots a day, I was put on a regimen of four shots a day to get the maximum control of blood sugar. Glucometers had recently been introduced in South Africa and I was encouraged to test myself routinely.

Unfortunately, I never did. It seemed like an enormous amount of unnecessary work, when I had always managed before without checking my blood sugar levels. The impending complications from diabetes and poor blood sugar control seemed a distant and strange concept when I was young. The need to find a happy medium between what was healthy and beneficial for me, and what would make me feel good, was always a struggle.

A physician once remarked on my skinniness, saying, "You don't want to be a model, do you?" And my immediate thoughts were: "Well why not? Why should I be limited in what I can be? Why can't I decide what I want to be?"

There was no flexibility in what that endocrinologist told me and what would be a peaceful and happy medium for me. Food and diabetes are interrelated and have a huge impact on one another. What I have come to realize is that support is key to long-term care.

Dr. Distiller recommended that I see his dietitian. This was the first time since my initial diagnosis that I had spoken to anyone about diet. Interestingly enough, the dietitian, Michelle, also had type 1 diabetes. It was an easy fit for us to discuss diet and the frustrations that go along with unexpected hypo or hyperglycemia, and how to manage it. I encourage everyone struggling with diet and stress management to seek out their very own "Michelle," who understands exactly what they are going through. As a health coach, I am able to guide my clients through both the nutrition aspect of treating their diabetes, as well as stress management and self-care through my "balance your blood sugar" program. Both are important aspects of managing diabetes.

After seeing Michelle, I made adjustments to my diet. I now had a better idea of food combinations and measurements to implement into my diet.

Healthy eating habits, as well as a healthy relationship with food is critical. Emotional wellbeing is also as essential as proper nutrition. Emotional hunger can lead to sabotage. It is vital to know why you are emotionally starved and how to meet those needs in order to be an emotionally-nourished, content and balanced person.

Chapter 2.

The Adventure Begins. USA, Here We Come!

Complications and Pregnancy

I have always felt as though people viewed me differently because I have type 1 diabetes. I felt that they found me to be flawed by it. I was afraid of rejection if I revealed too much too quickly.

I always attempted to appear "normal," without a care in the world. The truth is that you can never be carefree when you have a disease like type 1 diabetes. It stings emotionally wherever you go. There are no "vacations" from this chronic condition. It requires regular planning and attention. It is important to know when and what you will eat, when to check your blood sugar, and when to take your insulin shot.

Not eating a well-balanced diet regularly means you risk moments of shaking and sweating from hypoglycemia, or feeling nauseated and sluggish from hyperglycemia. Sometimes, you are not sure whether the sugar level is too high or too low, as the symptoms can be similar and it's difficult to differentiate between the two. It requires planning and always being prepared with a snack in case of emergency.

Telling Steve, my now husband of 31 years that I had diabetes was not an easy task. I felt that I was not being honest about who I was by not telling him. The first time I plucked up the courage to tell him I was a nervous wreck. We were on our third date and he reached over and took my hand in his, kissed it and said, "I know" in the gentlest way imaginable. I could have cried with relief. I knew then that he was a special human being who would love all of my imperfections.

Steve and I dated for a year before we married and I knew that I had found gold in him. While on our honeymoon in New York, we met up with my father's long-lost cousin. When my grandfather left Latvia, the family was split up. His siblings went to the United States and my grandfather went to South Africa. I recognized my relative immediately, because he not only had the same last name as my maiden name, but he also bore a strong resemblance to my father.

We were very keen to emigrate from South Africa due to the political uncertainty at the time. I had been working at St. Johns Eye Hospital, which was part of Baragwaneth Hospital in Soweto, as an eye therapist for several years. Traveling and working there became unsafe due to riots and stone throwing at passing cars.

My uncle secured job positions and willing sponsors in the US for us both, and three years later we immigrated to New Jersey. We were thrilled. We felt as though the world was at our feet as we moved on to a new and exciting chapter of our lives.

In the meantime, both my brother and sister had immigrated to Melbourne, Australia. My parents were to soon follow them. South Africa no longer felt like home to me without my family there.

During my first year of marriage, at 27 years old, I experienced my first diabetic complication. After seeing the same ophthalmologist, Basil Cummings, MD, in Johannesburg for several years without any problems, there was evidence of diabetic retinopathy in both my eyes.

"Chronically high blood sugar from diabetes is associated with damage to the tiny blood vessels in the retina, leading to diabetic retinopathy. Diabetic retinopathy can cause blood vessels in the retina to leak fluid or bleed, distorting vision. In its most advanced stage, new abnormal blood vessels increase in number on the surface of the retina, which can lead to scarring and cell loss in the retina.

For decades, PDR has been treated with scatter laser surgery, sometimes called panretinal laser surgery or panretinal photocoagulation. Treatment involves making tiny laser burns in areas of the retina away from the macula. These laser burns are intended to cause abnormal blood vessels to shrink. Several sessions of laser treatment may be necessary. While it can preserve central vision, laser surgery may cause some loss of side (peripheral), color, and night vision."[4]

If left untreated, diabetic retinopathy can lead to blindness and extensive laser surgery in both eyes was necessary for me.

It felt like a sharp sting of an elastic band. The closer to the perimeter of the retina, the more painful it became. The intensity and the brightness of the lamp made it difficult to keep the eye open while the laser was in progress.

Both eyes received laser treatment over a period of several weeks. Each session lasted about an hour, while the laser sealed the spot on the retina with the leaking vessel, preventing it from further bleeding. One eye is worked on at a time, and then given time to recover due to subsequent edema and tenderness. The vision also needed time to settle, before continuing treatment, until all the bleeding vessels were treated.

When I first received laser treatment and was able to fully process the extent of the detrimental effects of type 1 diabetes, I was in a state of shock. I developed intense migraines and had to be hospitalized and given morphine intravenously for the extreme pain. The stress of it created tension in my neck and shoulders, which required weeks of physical therapy.

The laser treatments proved to be highly successful and I am forever grateful to Basil Cummings, MD who

4   National Eye Institute, Facts about Diabetic Eye Disease: Sept, 2015: http//nei.nih.gov/health/diabetic/retinopathy

did a remarkable job of saving my vision. Because of him, I still maintain excellent vision in each eye.

Over the next several years, I still needed more laser treatments, but none affected me to quite the same extent as that initial diagnosis of diabetic retinopathy. This opened up a whole new level of stress and concern for me. It made me realize that I was not immune to the diabetic complications that I had feared, and that it was my responsibility to take control of my blood sugar levels before it was too late. Most newlyweds do not concern themselves with major health issues, however, our marriage suddenly took on a whole new dimension of concern.

I had consulted with an obstetrician in South Africa about having children, and was told that under no circumstance would I ever be able to conceive or carry a child. Conception for a diabetic woman can be difficult, and tight control of blood sugar is necessary for months previous to conception. The news was completely devastating. I couldn't accept the fact that having children was not in the cards for us. What he didn't tell me was that with hard work, and with a good medical team specializing in high-risk pregnancies, it was possible.

Despite all the warnings, six months after emigration, I got pregnant. We were ecstatic. We couldn't believe how fortunate we were, particularly after hearing that I would not be able to conceive. I was determined to do everything within my power to ensure delivery of a healthy baby.

Although getting pregnant was relatively easy, the pregnancy itself proved to be the opposite. Pregnancy for most women can be challenging even without diabetes in the equation, but for women with type 1 diabetes, the pressure to do everything "right" is compounded. My blood sugars had not been in a desirable range before conception, which added to the complexity of doing everything possible to ensure a healthy baby.

My baby thrived but I had a tough time stabilizing my blood sugar and keeping it under tight control. I became good friends with my glucometer, and tested many times a day, due to the dramatic and unexpected fluctuations that occur during pregnancy.

The first trimester passed fairly uneventfully and Steve and I were delighted with my expanding belly. All the tests were normal and the pregnancy, as well as my developing baby, was progressing beautifully. We took such pleasure and delight in planning for the birth of our child.

I resigned from my job at the doctor's office four months into the pregnancy. I was informed by both my endocrinologist and obstetrician that I would need to devote all my time and energy to maintaining steady, normal blood sugar levels in order to ensure a healthy pregnancy and baby. Following doctors' orders became my full-time focus and occupation.

Interestingly, no one addressed the nutritional aspect of the pregnancy with me. I stayed off caffeine, but besides that, ate much the same as I had always eaten, instinctively making sure I ate plenty of fresh fruit and vegetables and adequate protein.

I highly recommend working with a health coach or

nutritionist during pregnancy to make sure that you are eating a nutrient dense diet that is nourishing and safe for both the mother and the baby.

During my first trimester, we spent a weekend in the Catskill Mountains. Besides feeling nauseated in the mornings, I felt quite well and energized, and we went for long hikes in the mountains.

Self-care and keeping physically active is an important aspect of a healthy pregnancy, particularly when you have diabetes, in order to maintain steady blood sugar levels.

Steve and I joined a health club that was near where we lived so that I could remain active throughout the pregnancy. I tested my blood sugar levels feverishly throughout the day to make adjustments accordingly.

Blood sugar levels can fluctuate dramatically during the second trimester.

One weekend, while we were exercising, I felt weak and shaky, and had blurred vision during an exercise class. I sat down at a table to test my blood sugar, and as I took out my glucometer and attempted to do a finger stick, I slipped to the floor. Steve saw what was happening and immediately ran for help. There were several physicians at the health club who suggested orange juice and an ambulance but refused to be involved any further.

I was taken by ambulance to Overlook Hospital in Summit, NJ. My blood sugar slowly stabilized while I was in the emergency room. It was a terrifying experience for both of us.

That incident was to be the first of many trips to the emergency room throughout our lives. We worried about harm to the baby because of the very low blood sugar levels. Thankfully, both the baby and I were unscathed by the experience.

During the second trimester, I woke up one morning and could not see with my right eye. I had just seen a new endocrinologist in New York City by the name of Andrew Drexler, MD, who immediately got me an appointment with Stanley Chang, MD, a retinal surgeon in New York City, specializing in diabetic retinopathy.

It turned out that I had a retinal detachment and needed more laser treatments to stop any further bleeding, as well as to repair the detachment. I was instructed to sleep upright and cover my right eye with a patch. The panic and stress was exacerbated by the fact that I was pregnant and needed my vision not only for myself, but also for my unborn child.

After several treatments, the blood began to clear, and I was able to see again with my right eye. Once the edema settled, besides a few more blind spots in my peripheral vision, my vision stabilized, and I felt like I was back to normal.

On reaching the third trimester, my blood pressure began to rise considerably and I was hospitalized and put on permanent bed rest. My uncle, being a member of the board of directors of Overlook Hospital, secured me a private room with a magnificent view of the green foliage outside. This was my only glimpse of summer, which was a blessing since I remained there for five full weeks, bloated miserable and scared, until my baby was born.

My parents arrived from Australia to help, and walked to the hospital every day to visit me and keep my spirits high. With the fluid retention, and the spike in blood pressure, I developed toxemia and preeclampsia, a condition that can lead to convulsions and coma, made worse by diabetes.

The obstetrician was waiting anxiously for my baby's lungs to develop sufficiently to proceed with a C-section. Gabrielle was born in July 1988. She was a beautiful, healthy baby girl, born a month premature, and weighed in at eight pounds and four ounces. This was not uncommon as diabetic moms generally deliver slightly bigger babies. But most importantly—she was healthy.

In no time at all, she was in the regular nursery, out of the intensive care unit, and the darling of all the nursing staff.

After 2 days Gaby was moved out of the neonatal intensive care unit. I, on the other hand, was immediately sent to intensive care unit, with fluid on my lungs and heart from the toxemia. My blood pressure had soared through the roof and my head felt as though it would explode. I drifted in and out of consciousness and begged Steve not to leave me. I was terrified that I would slip away. Gaby and I finally met the next day once I was stabilized.

I cradled her in my arms for a few precious moments, while still hooked up to beeping monitors and an IV.

She was so adorable and perfect in every way. As I held her, with tears streaming down my face, I thanked God for making me the luckiest woman in the world. Suddenly everything changed. My child needed me and was counting on me to be well and take care of her for years to come.

I fed her for the first time, before she was taken back to the nursery. My obstetrician then arrived and informed me in no uncertain terms that this was to be both my first and last pregnancy.

I felt unfazed by his advice, as I had just held and fed my perfect baby girl.

A year after Gaby was born, the movie Steel Magnolias, was released into cinemas around the country. For those unfamiliar with the film, Shelby, played by Julia Roberts, is a type 1 diabetic who, due to her disease, had very weak kidney function. She was advised by her doctor not to have children, but wanted a child so badly that she got pregnant anyway. The strain of pregnancy and childbirth put her into kidney failure. Her mother donated a kidney to her; however, unfortunately Shelby rejected it and died at the end of the film. [5]

---

5   *Steel Magnolias.* Dir. Herbert Ross. Perf. Sally Field, Dolly Parton, Julia Roberts, Daryl Hannah, Olympia Dukakis, Shirley MacLaine, Tom Skerritt, and Sam Shepard. Tri-Star, 1989.

Chapter 3

Diabetic Dietary Recommendations

It was Hippocrates who said, "Let food be thy medicine and medicine be thy food." Blood sugar levels can be maintained at a healthy level by choosing the right food combinations and portion sizes, exercising regularly and managing/taking care of emotional health the best you can.

This is easier said than done, as blood sugar management can be like walking a tightrope and with that—an emotional rollercoaster. But it is important to regularly check your blood sugar levels and know how to regulate them and eat accordingly.

Knowing your average blood sugar level is a vital step of managing your type 1 diabetes. This can be measured by a hemoglobin A1c test. The test is a measure of your blood sugar control over the past two to three months. The goal is to have an A1c test below seven percent. A result of eight percent or more is a sign that changes need to be made to better manage blood sugar levels.

Why is managing blood sugar level so important?

The findings of the Diabetes Control and Complications Trial (DCCT)7 have shown that people with diabetes who manage their blood sugar levels well, with A1c levels close to seven percent can delay the onset or potentially prevent diabetes-related complications that affect the eyes, kidneys and nerves.

Ideally your blood sugar level should be between 80-130 mg/dl before mealtimes and less than180 mg/dl one to two hours after a meal.

Diabetes Superfoods

Below is a list of the top diabetes superfoods to include in your diet. Before making any changes to your diet, it is advisable to first consult your dietitian or physician. I suggest working out meal plans and menus with a dietitian or health coach in order to make a healthful diet that balances your blood sugar level, part of your daily regimen.

As with all foods, you need to include superfoods into your particular meal plan in appropriate portions, focusing on combining proteins, fats and carbohydrates in every meal. Your plate should be three quarters green leafy vegetables and the remaining quarter, protein the size of a deck of cards, and a small amount of unrefined low glycemic index carbohydrates. The glycemic index (GI) is the ranking of carbohydrate-containing foods, based on the food's total effect on blood glucose. It is important to ration the amount of carbohydrates that you eat in each meal,with a target not to exceed

15 grams per meal. As with most diet plans, there is no one size that fits all, it is bio individual depending on age, gender, and activity level. Getting fiber from plant foods, such as whole grains, fruits, vegetables, beans and nuts will help balance your blood sugar and slow down the process of absorption of carbohydrates into the blood stream.

All non-fiber carbohydrates break down into sugar and it's important to read labels correctly and calculate the amount of carbohydrates that you consume per serving. To count the net carbohydrates, consider the serving size and the carbohydrate value. Deduct the amount of fiber from the carbohydrates and you will get the net carbohydrate value. Divide this by 15 to evaluate how many portions of carbohydrate per serving size.

Make your plate a rainbow of colors to pack in as many macro (carbohydrates, protein and fat) and micro (vitamins and minerals) nutrients as possible.

Healthy fats, such as olive oil, avocado oil or nuts, are also an essential part of each meal. It is advisable to eat six small meals per day, as opposed to three, to keep blood sugar levels stable and to eat ahead of your hunger. This keeps you satiated for longer, without spikes in blood sugar or hypoglycemic emergencies. A single fat serving size is usually one to two teaspoons of unsaturated fats per meal, one and a half teaspoons of nut butter, or two tablespoons of avocado.

The superfoods in the list below have a low-glycemic index and are perfect for a diabetic-friendly diet. They provide key nutrients that are lacking in the standard American diet, better known as the SAD diet, such as calcium, potassium, fiber, magnesium and vitamins A, C and E.

Always target getting your nutrients from food, as there is no research that definitively shows that supplementation is a better choice for vitamin and mineral sources.

Protein

Whole organic eggs, wild fish (salmon, grouper, black cod), grass fed beef and organic free range poultry are all good options. A serving should be the size of your palm, or a deck of cards. Protein is essential for building muscle tissue in the body. If taken with carbohydrates, fat and fiber, protein will be digested and released into the blood stream and cells at a slower rate. Protein also optimizes your brain's ability to send messages to the rest of your body and keeps you energized. However, consuming too much protein is not beneficial, as excess protein is stored as fat.

Beans

Navy, pinto, kidney and black beans all provide wonderful nutrition. They all have a high fiber content and nourish you with about one third of your daily requirement of protein in just one half of a cup, without the saturated fat. They are also good sources of magnesium and potassium. Canned beans can act as a readily available source of protein, but make sure to drain and rinse them to reduce the sodium content. As with most foods, organic beans are best. They serve as a carbohydrate source as well as a protein source, so be sure to calculate that into your diet plan.

Dark Green Leafy Vegetables

Powerhouse foods like spinach, collards, bok choy, kale, cabbage, onions, Brussels sprouts and green beans are low in calories, packed with fiber (which helps stabilize blood sugar) and have a low GI carbohydrate. Dark leafy greens, such as kale, boost the immune system and help strengthen the respiratory and blood systems. Try and rotate the greens you eat to achieve maximum benefits. I prefer to get my carbohydrates in vegetable form and avoid the highly-processed and refined carbohydrates that are addictive and rapidly absorbed into the bloodstream. Leafy greens are packed with calcium, magnesium, iron, phosphorous, zinc and vitamins A, C and K. Green vegetables also help replenish our alkaline mineral store and filter out toxins and pollutants. Try and eat at least two to three servings of greens per day. A serving size is usually one half a cup cooked, or one cup raw, and should comprise three quarters of the real estate on your plate.

Citrus Fruit

Grapefruit, lemons, oranges and limes are loaded with soluble fiber and vitamin C, and are lower GI fruits. A serving of fruit, usually one small orange or a half a grapefruit, is a great source of carbohydrate.

Sweet Potatoes

These are starchy vegetables dense in vitamin A and fiber. Substitute them in place of regular potatoes for a lower GI carbohydrate alternative. A half a cup is the usual serving size, or one quarter of the plate.

Berries

Blueberries, strawberries, raspberries, and black-berries are all packed full of antioxidants, vitamins and fiber, and are very low-glycemic fruits. A serving size is three quarters to a cup of berries per serving. Make sure they are organic, as berries are packed with pesticide residue.

Tomatoes

Whether your tomatoes are pureed, raw, or in a sauce, they are full of vital nutrients like vitamin C, iron and vitamin E. The lycopene found in tomatoes is a very powerful antioxidant, which helps to protect body cells from harmful free radicals.

Fish High in Omega-3 Fatty Acid

Wild caught salmon is a great choice in this category. Smaller fish contain less mercury, so opt for sardines, herring, trout, grouper and seafood such as shrimp, mussels, crab and clams.

Whole Grains

The germ and bran of the whole grain contain all the nutrients a grain product has to offer. Processed foods like bread made from enriched wheat flour, don't have any of these nutrients. Whole grains also provide fiber, potassium, magnesium, chromium, omega three fatty acids, and folate. It has been found that most people with an autoimmune disease, such as diabetes, Lupus, Hashimoto's or any other autoimmune disease, do better on a gluten free diet.[6] According to Amy Myers, author of "*The Autoimmune Solution: Prevent and Reverse the Full Spectrum of Inflammatory Symptoms and Diseases,*" continued use of gluten aggravates these situations. Try to opt for gluten free options when it comes to grains, such as quinoa, brown rice, amaranth and teff." Avoid processed breads and other processed products, as they are loaded with sugar and preservatives. You can purchase gluten free oats, which are made in a dedicated facility, so they are not contaminated by regular oats.

Nuts

An ounce of nuts provides key healthy fats. A portion of nuts is also great for hunger management. Other benefits of nuts are a healthy dose of magnesium and fiber. Additionally, some nuts and seeds, such as walnuts and flax seeds, are a great source of omega-3 fatty acids.

---

6   Amy Myers, The Autoimmune Solution: Prevent and Reverse the Full Spectrum of Inflammatory Symptoms and Diseases– January 27, 2015

Healthy Fats

These are an essential part of a low carbohydrate diet, as they help you feel satisfied and are used as the a primary source of fuel. Good options are olive oil, coconut oil, sesame oil, nut butters, avocado and grass fed butter or ghee.

Milk and Yogurt

Dairy can help build strong bones and teeth as it contains calcium. Many fortified dairy products are also a good source of vitamin D. There is a lot of evidence on the connection between vitamin D and good health.

Chapter 4.

Kidney and Pancreas Transplant

Life seemed to be an ongoing series of challenges. Growing up and coping with type 1 diabetes and trying to hide the fact that I was different from other children was difficult.

As an adolescent and young adult, I felt unable to be carefree and struggled to open up to others, as most people of my age did. After I got married and had my daughter, I was afraid of driving and getting involved in activities with her in case I had a low blood sugar, as I would have to pull off the road and couldn't tend to her adequately. Highway driving became a nightmare. It made me feel inadequate and out of control. Later on, as I managed to conquer these fears and manage my diabetes, I began to contemplate my first transplant, a double organ kidney and pancreas transplant.

Soon after Gaby was born, I was informed that I would need to have a transplant in approximately seven years' time, as my kidneys were regressing. Both diabetes and the preeclampsia during pregnancy had taken their toll on my kidneys. I was horrified. I had seen how disabling dialysis was, and how it left people feeling sick and weak.

There were no guarantees that dialysis would keep me alive indefinitely, should it come to that. Additionally, I wondered if I would be strong enough to withstand a transplant. I also worried about the possibility that my body would reject the transplanted organs, and I would not survive the surgery.

I had radically reduced the protein intake, as well as potassium and phosphorous in my diet. I did so to try to preserve my kidneys for as long as possible in order to delay going on dialysis. A nutritionist or health coach with expertise in dietary recommendations for someone with insufficient kidney function would have been a great help during this time. I somehow managed with the help of a very experienced nurse practitioner, and by doing my own research, to figure it out.

But sure enough, seven years after Gaby was born, Steve and I flew to the University Of Minnesota Hospital where we consulted David Sutherland, MD, a world renowned transplant surgeon and the pioneer of the double organ, kidney and pancreas transplant surgery.

In October 1994, I was told that it might be a long wait, but amazingly, five months later, I received a call confirming that they had organs for me.

I felt paralyzed with shock and fear.

We immediately started planning how to get to

Minnesota by the next available flight, as being a cadaver donor, time was of the essence. We arrived in the afternoon with seven year old Gaby in tow. After a tense flight, we immediately proceeded to the hospital. On our arrival, I was prepared for surgery and taken to the operating room without wasting time. The donor was a perfect match, and given that I had antibodies from pregnancy, the urgency of the procedure was tenfold.

I explained to Gaby that after the surgery I would not need to take shots every day or check my blood sugar regularly. She was delighted with this piece of information and exclaimed, "You won't need shots anymore, you will be all better. I am so happy!" My fear dissipated at her happiness and innocence and with that I resolved to go on with the surgery.

After a nine-hour-long surgery and many hours of waiting, Steve and Gaby finally got some sleep and rest. They were assured that the surgery was successful. The recovery was a long and slow process. The pancreas is a very delicate organ that requires a long adjustment period. But after a short while, I was completely off insulin shots and relying on my new functioning pancreas to secrete insulin. The kidney was also functioning well. The recovery from the actual procedure took a whole year. I remained in the hospital for a month. Steve and Gaby stayed in Minnesota for two weeks, and Gaby once more became the darling of all the nurses. She was a ray of shining light for me and remained my inspiration throughout my long and arduous recovery.

There was a huge window looking out onto the

courtyard at the end of the transplant wing where Gaby drew a beautiful rainbow, with a pot of gold at the end of it, with crayons given to her to keep her busy. I soon realized the significance of what she had drawn. Every time I walked by, it would bring comfort and joy to me, even after Gaby went back to New Jersey to attend school.

After I returned home, I was told by Gaby's second-grade teacher that she had asked the children to describe their most special day. Most children spoke about birthday parties, cake, and toys. Gaby told her classmates, "My most special day was when my mom came home from the hospital."

Not having any immediate family in the U.S., my sister Bonita and her six year old daughter Leigh came from Melbourne, Australia and stayed with us for several weeks. Bonita took care of Steve, Gaby and me, as I continued with my recovery process.

Two weeks after returning home, I was rushed back to Minnesota after developing pancreatitis. This is a disease in which the pancreas becomes inflamed, causing severe pain, nausea and vomiting. I was put on bed rest and taken off food and liquid until the pancreatitis subsided. I was then able to tolerate a regular diet again.

By the time I came home, Bonita and Leigh had gone back to Australia. I was devastated that I had not been able to say good-bye to them, and that they had left with the impression that I was not doing better with my recovery. The void of not having close family nearby seemed greater than ever as I slowly recovered from this life changing surgery. It took more than a year before I was able to visit my family in Australia.

The most difficult adjustment for me post-transplant was taking all the medications that I needed to keep the transplanted organs functioning. I felt completely overwhelmed by the quantity of medications as well as the regularity with which I had to take them. I was on a regimen of taking meds four times daily, which seemed incredibly arduous. But as I began to recover, it became easier.

Initially, I took three different anti-rejection medications, as well as blood pressure meds among others. The anti-rejection meds were slowly titrated to a maintenance dosage. I did lab work once a week to gauge the health of the kidney and pancreas. As time progressed, I was able to cut back to checking lab work every other week, and finally after six months, to once a month.

As I adjusted to my new regimen and identity, I began to enjoy life with a new freedom that I had never previously known. If I was not hungry, I did not have to eat, and if I wanted dessert, that was okay too.

For so many years I had identified myself as a "diabetic," so it felt both foreign and strange to think and behave differently. I still consider myself a type 1 diabetic. I feel as though being a diabetic has been intricately woven into the fabric of both my identity and DNA. However, I also always view myself as a three-dimensional person, and not only as someone who has type 1 diabetes. It is important to note that my new freedom was achieved through great physical and emotional cost.

To celebrate the first anniversary post-transplant, I took a trip to Paris and Provence to drink in this new found freedom. It made me sad to see young people having fun, without the thoughts of illness and mortality that I had been saddled with for most of my life. But at the same time, I was so grateful for the gift of life, and freedom from regular testing of blood sugar and insulin shots.

I arrived home feeling blessed and elated, ready to take on the world and enjoy life to the fullest with my family.

Chapter 5.

Search for a Kidney and Dialysis

I enjoyed good health for ten wonderful years, and was able to live an active and full life as a wife, mother and member of the community. I worked for a pediatric ophthalmologist for several years, until our family moved to Atlanta, Georgia.

During this period, we celebrated my 40th birthday, Gaby's Bat Mitzvah, and Steve's 50th. Career opportunities for Steve required us to move interstate several times. Our first move happened a year after the transplant. We moved from New Jersey to Jacksonville, Florida. After four years, we then returned to New Jersey for a three-year stint, before relocating to Atlanta, Georgia for 11 years. The relocation proved to be challenging for both Gaby and me. Each relocation not only necessitated finding a new community and new friends but also a new group of doctors to coordinate my care. It takes a village right?

After our relocation to Atlanta, we bought a house. Gaby was finally well settled in high school and busy with SATs and college applications. All in all, life seemed pretty great.

I felt particularly sluggish following a trip from Israel. My serum creatinine level, a marker of kidney function had begun creeping up, which alarmed my nephrologist, Antonio Guasch, MD, at Emory Hospital.

Due to repeated urinary tract infections, the only treatment option for me was an enteric conversion, whereby the transplanted pancreas would be hooked up to the small intestine, instead of the bladder. The surgery was done at The University of Minnesota Medical School where I had the kidney and pancreas transplant. After the surgery, which proved to be a mammoth procedure, the urinary tract infections improved, but the stress of the surgery had an adverse effect on the transplanted kidney.

The recovery took months. I experienced regular nausea and body weakening. I was unable to eat and enjoy food without vomiting. I lost a tremendous amount of weight in a relatively short period of time. I spent endless weeks in bed, unable to function and attend to daily family needs and issues. I have a distinct memory of the sadness I saw in Steve and Gaby's faces, while they were seeing me so ill and trapped in bed. I was not able to be the wife or the mother I had always strived to be, and was incapable of fully sharing in daily highs and lows of family living. The result was not what I had hoped for, after such an enormous and invasive surgery.

Steve was immediately tested to see if he could be a match for me for a second kidney transplant. He returned from the test in tears confirming that we were not a match. We began searching to find a compatible kidney for me.

Desperate to end the nightmare that I was facing, we looked in every direction and followed every possible lead in our search for a compatible kidney. I was first listed at the University of Minnesota after the enteric conversion. The other hospital I was listed at was Emory University Hospital, where I received all my care. Both hospitals confirmed that the wait would be approximately two to three years.

On April 5th 2006, I had my first dialysis treatment. This date will forever be embedded in my memory as one of the toughest days of my life. My fear and horror of my journey leading to this event had always lurked in my subconscious mind as a far off possibility. I had always held on to the childish belief that I would be spared this hardship. The day before my first hemodialysis treatment, a temporary port with two plastic tubes was surgically inserted into my upper right chest. This permanent catheter was a tube inserted into a vein, with two attached tubes or chambers to allow a two-way flow of blood. The dialysis needles were then placed into each outlet—one to take the blood out of my body and cleanse it, and the other to feed the blood back into my body once it was free of toxins. Once a catheter was placed, it was not necessary to use a needle for intravenous access. Unfortunately, these permanent catheters are known to clog easily and cause infection and narrowing of the vein where they are attached.

This was not a permanent solution for access. It was essential for me to keep it dry and sterile for months until permanent access could be surgically placed in my upper arm.

I was wheeled into the dialysis room at Emory University Hospital with bright artificial lights and enormous dialysis machines buzzing and beeping.

The patients were lying and murmuring as if in pain—each at a different point of completion of treatment. I felt as though I had entered into an unfamiliar world—one that I had no control over, and had no wish to be a part of. I felt helpless, horrified and trapped. One young girl was crying out in pain as a nurse was trying to put the dialysis needles into her AV graft. I wondered with dread whether it was going to be painful for me too.

After being hooked up to the machine, I began to relax. It did not feel as bad as it appeared, and my fears were temporarily allayed. "If this is all it is, I can do this," I thought.

The treatment lasted three hours, during which time I used visualization and deep breathing to put myself into a meditative state and help myself get through that initial fear and release stress. Once it was done, I was taken back to my hospital room to rest—mentally and physically exhausted. After my first introduction to hemodialysis, I had no idea that the procedure would dictate the framework of my existence for the next two years.

I felt trapped in so many ways: Trapped by the dependence on dialysis; trapped in my house after each and every dialysis treatment that left me feeling weak and drained and unable to get out of bed; stuck in Atlanta, unable to visit Gaby in college out of state without arranging for dialysis, and unable to visit my family in Australia; and trapped by all my fear and anxiety of never being able to live a normal life again.

After coming home from Emory Hospital with a few dialysis treatments under my belt as an inpatient, arrangements were made for me to see a dialysis nephrologist and have my treatments done at his clinic. I had to schedule appointments three days a week and wait for a machine to be available. The technician would then prepare me, insert the needles into my permanent catheter, and hook me up for my three-hour ordeal.

The initial horror of the dialysis clinic became a regular trial for me. Listening to everyone's stories, I became more and more withdrawn and depressed, without hope of a change to my fate. The constant drone of the machines, combined with the beeping when fluids needed replacement and patients crying out, was too much to bear.

Thankfully, we were able to make arrangements for me to have the next series of dialysis treatments at home, with little to no extra additional cost to us. Our insurance also covered the cost of a visiting nurse to administer and monitor the treatment, as well as the use of the machine. We had the dialysis machine installed in our spare bedroom.

I needed to have surgery to have a fistula inserted to replace the permanent catheter. However, unbeknown to us, my veins were too fragile and insubstantial to withstand a fistula and I underwent two failed attempts at fistula surgeries in my left wrist and forearm.

For those unfamiliar with this treatment, an AV fistula is surgically created to connect a vein and an artery, typically in the arm. This is the access created routinely for hemodialysis. This type of hemodialysis access is the least likely kind of vascular access to form clots or become infected. By connecting the artery to the vein, more blood flows to the vein and it becomes stronger, making repeated needle insertions easier. However, after the two failed attempts, a synthetic graft, the only remaining option, was placed in my upper left arm.

A dialysis graft is made by connecting an artery to a vein by inserting a plastic tube, which then becomes an artificial vein under the skin. This can then be repeatedly used for needle placement and blood access during hemodialysis. A graft does not take the time to develop, as a fistula does, and can be used two to three weeks after insertion, as opposed to a fistula that may take months to develop. The downside of AV graft is that it has more problems with clotting and infection, and often needs replacement.

I continued undergoing dialysis in the comfort of my home, experiencing many side effects caused by dialysis.

Sometimes my blood pressure would be too low, causing consequent nausea, throwing up and severe cramping. There were also frequent unexpected disasters during this time. For instance, out of the blue, I would be ready to undergo a dialysis treatment, feeling uncomfortable and bloated with fluid and my AV graft would be blocked. I would need to be rushed to the emergency room to have it surgically unblocked.

I became regular at the Emory Radiology center, where they would say, "Oh Ms. Zunde, you are back again!" as they struggled to find a vein for the IV. Finding an adequate vein was always a challenge. It often took three to four painful attempts before locating it.

However, the pain was of no concern when compared to the success of the procedure. The relief I felt once the AV graft was open, and I could resume dialysis and the nightmare existence that had become my life, was enormous.

This routine went on for two agonizing years. I became more frail and weak with each passing week of dialysis treatments. I also started experiencing terrible chills, accompanied by nausea and vomiting. In addition, the site of the permanent catheter appeared to be infected, but no one could figure out what type of infection it was.

Eventually, my dermatologist took a biopsy and discovered that it was not an infection at all, but Proliferative Transplant Lymphoma (PTLD). This was caused by the immunosuppressant drugs that I had been taking since the first transplant in 1995. So sadly, I became a cancer patient on top of being a dialysis patient. The oncologist assigned to me was Leonard Heffner, MD, a real Southern gentleman. He treated me in the kindest, most respectful way, and I am forever grateful to him. The course of treatment was four infusions of Rituxan over a four-week period. I had dialysis on Tuesdays, Thursdays and Saturdays, while on Wednesdays I went to the oncology clinic at Emory to receive the Rituxin.

Going to an oncology unit was the most humbling experience. As miserable as I felt, I only had to look at the people having treatments nearby—many old and young alike with four or five different cocktails mixed into their IVs.

Fortunately, the Rituxan treatments proved successful and I only had to deal with dialysis for the next year. I impatiently held on to the hope that at the end, I would be considered healthy enough to have a transplant.

While I was recovering from the treatments, my sister brought my 76-year-old mother from Australia to visit me for one precious week. My mom was riddled with arthritis and taking care of my 87-year-old father, who was suffering from heart failure and dementia. Determined to visit me, my mother placed my dad in respite care in Australia. I was so excited and happy to have both my sister and mom in my home. It had been almost 10 years since my parents had visited us in the US.

I cherished this time with them, soaking up their unconditional love and devotion, while mindful of the lengths they had gone to be with me. The time flew by in the blink of an eye.

Several days into their visit, I received a call from the University of Minnesota Hospital confirming that they had a kidney for me. I tearfully informed the hospital that I had just finished Rituxan treatment for lymphoma and asked if it was still possible for me to have the transplant. Needless to say, their response was negative. I had to wait at least a year to ensure there was no recurrence of lymphoma, before I could once again be a transplant candidate.

Consumed with disappointment and emotion, I broke down sobbing, uncontrollably. The weight of my situation came crashing down on me. This was the first glimpse at healthy life and I was unable to embrace it.

Our next obstacle was to find a transplant center that would put me on their waiting list, as I had been removed from all the lists I was on previously, following the Lymphoma diagnosis. I was considered a risky candidate for a kidney transplant, with a questionable life expectancy.

To quote statistics, more than 3,000 new patients are added to the kidney waiting list each month, and 13 people die each day while waiting for a life-saving kidney transplant.[7] The odds were stacked against us, but that did not stop us from continuing our search.

During this time, a friend called to give us the contact details of a man who had undergone two kidney transplants in New York City. We immediately arranged for me to have dialysis there so we could talk to him and learn how he had achieved this feat. Steve booked a hotel and flights—and off we went, full of hope and determination to contact anyone that could help us end our nightmare.

---

7   NKF, 2015 http://optn.transplant.hrsa.gov/

We met the elusive religious man at a kosher restaurant in New York City. Steve, Gaby and I sat, hopeful and eager while he told us about his experiences. However, he failed to address the purpose of our meeting. As we finished our lunch, we had not yet learned how to speed up the process of finding a kidney, until Steve reminded him of why we were there. He then scribbled three potential hospitals on a piece of paper and left. There was no divine intervention or solution to our problem. There was no quick fix to finding a kidney for me. We were left feeling disappointed and distraught. Our search for a kidney continued.

We then placed an urgent call for hope to the local Jewish newspaper in Atlanta. They wrote a story about our plight. Since I have A positive blood, I was a potential match with anyone with type O or type A positive blood. The article explained how we had sought a match from family members in both South Africa and Australia, but had been unsuccessful. The contact details at Emory University Hospital were included, but nobody called. Meanwhile, I was getting weaker as the weeks went by.

Chapter 6

Dietary Requirements While on Dialysis

While on dialysis, I learn't about following a low potassium, low phosphorus and low protein diet. It is necessary to reduce these minerals and macronutrients if your kidneys do not function properly.

According to the National Kidney Foundation, the following is a guideline as to what to eat and limit while on dialysis (or just prior) to put minimal stress on the kidneys and the body. It is advisable to keep this list handy because potassium is present in so many sources and the diet tends to be counterintuitive.

A kidney-friendly diet may also help limit certain minerals in the foods you eat. This helps keep waste from building up in your blood and may help prevent other health problems.

Potassium is a mineral found in many of the foods you eat. It plays a role in keeping your heartbeat regular and your muscles working correctly. Healthy kidneys maintain the correct amount of potassium in your body.

However, when your kidneys are not healthy, it is vital to limit certain foods that increase potassium levels in your blood. You can experience weakness, numbness and tingling if your potassium is too high, which may cause an irregular heartbeat or a heart attack.[8]

You should check with your doctor about your monthly blood potassium level. If it is lower than 3.5-5.0, you are in the safe zone. If it is 5.1-6.0, you are in the caution zone, and if it is higher than 6.0, you are in the danger zone.

Below are tips for keeping potassium from getting too high:

- Limit high potassium foods. A renal dietitian can help you plan your diet so you can get the correct amount of potassium.

- Eat a variety of foods in moderation.

- Leach high potassium foods, if you want to include them in your diet. Leaching is a process that pulls potassium out of the vegetables.

Leaching

The process of leaching helps pull some of the potassium out of high potassium vegetables. It is important to know that it does not pull all the potassium out, so you still need to limit the amount you consume. Check

---

[8]   National Kidney Foundation, 2015 https://www.kidney.org

with your dietician about how much of these leached vegetables you can safely eat.

Leaching vegetables

- Slice vegetables 1/8 inch thick.

- Rinse in warm water for a few seconds.

- Soak for a minimum of two hours in warm water. Use 10 times the amount of water to the amount of vegetables. If soaking longer, change the water every four hours.

- Rinse again under warm water for several seconds.

- Cook vegetable with five times the amount of water to the amount of vegetable.

- Check with your renal dietitian on the amount of leached vegetables to safely include in your diet.

- Do not use the liquid from canned fruits and vegetables, or juice from cooked meat.

- Remember that most foods have potassium. The serving size is critical. Large amounts of low potassium food become high potassium foods.

- If you are on dialysis, be sure to get all treatments and exchanges prescribed to you.

The correct amount of potassium intake per day on a potassium restricted diet is typically 2,000 mg per day.

A renal dietitian will help you make modifications to prevent complications for kidney disease. The portion size is ½ cup, or 200 mg of potassium, unless otherwise stated. It is important to check portion sizes, as some foods are higher in potassium than others.

High Potassium Foods

Fruits	Vegetables
2 Apricots raw, or 5 dried	Acorn Squash
Avocado, ¼ whole	Artichoke
Banana, ½ whole	Bamboo Shoots
Cantaloupe	Baked Beans
Dates, 5 whole	Butternut Squash
Dried fruits	Refried beans
Figs, dried	Beets, fresh, then boiled
Grapefruit juice	Black beans
Honeydew	Broccoli, cooked
Kiwi, 1 medium	Brussels sprouts
Mango, 1 medium	Chinese cabbage
Nectarine, 1 medium	Carrots
Orange, 1 medium	Dried beans
Orange juice	Greens, except kale

Fruits	Vegetables
Papaya, ½ whole	Hubbard squash
Pomegranates, 1 whole	Kohlrabi
Pomegranate juice	Lentils
Prune	Legumes
Prune juice	White mushrooms
Raisins	Okra
	Parsnips
	Potatoes, white
	Pumpkin
	Rutabagas
	Spinach,
	Tomato products
	Vegetable juices
Other Food	
All bran products	
Chocolate	
Milk products	
Molasses	
Nuts and seeds	
Peanut butter, 2 TB	
Salt free broth	
Yoghurt	

Remember, eating more than one serving can turn a lower potassium food into a high potassium food.

Low Potassium Foods

Fruits	Vegetables
Apple, 1 medium	Alfalfa Sprouts
Apple juice	Asparagus
Applesauce	Beans, green
Apricots, canned in juice	Broccoli
Blackberries	Celery
Blueberries	Cauliflower
Cherries	Corn, ½ ear
Cranberries	Cucumber
Fruit cocktail	Kale
Eggplant	Carrots
Grapes	Mixed Veg
Grape juice	White mushroom
Grapefruit, 1/2	Onions
Mandarins Oranges	Parsley
Peaches, fresh 1 small, Canned ½ cup	Peas, Green
	Peppers
Pears, 1 small fresh, ½ cup canned	Radish
	Rhubarb
Pineapple, and juice	Water chestnuts
Plums, 1 whole	Watercress
Raspberries	Yellow squash
Strawberries	Zucchini
Tangerine, 1 cup	
Watermelon, 1 cup	

Other Foods
Bread products, no whole grains
Coffee, 8 oz. limit
Cake, angel, yellow
Pasta
Pies without chocolate or fruit high in potassium
Noodles
Cookies, without nuts or chocolate
Rice
Tea, limit 16 oz.

What is Phosphorous?

According to the National Kidney Foundation, phosphorous is found in your bones. Along with calcium, phosphorus is needed for building healthy and strong bones, as well as keeping other parts of your body healthy.[9]

Normal functioning kidneys can remove extra phosphorus in your blood. When you have Chronic Kidney Disease, CKD, your kidneys cannot remove phosphorus efficiently. High phosphorous levels in your blood can cause damage to your body. Additional unused phosphorous causes changes in your body that pull the calcium from your bones, weakening them. High phosphorous and calcium levels also lead to dangerous calcium deposits in blood vessels, lungs, eyes, and heart. It is imperative to control both calcium and phosphorous levels for overall health.

9　NKF, 2015 https://www.kidney.org/about/contact

A normal phosphorus level is 2.5-4.5 mg/Dl. To maintain good phosphorous levels, it is necessary to understand your diet. Your dietitian and doctor will help with this.

The following is a list of foods high in phosphorous to limit or avoid.

Beverages	
Ale	Beer
Cocoa	Chocolate drinks
Dark soda	Milk drinks
Canned iced tea	
Dairy Products	
Cheese	Ice cream
Cottage cheese	Cream soups
Custard	Yoghurt
Protein	
Carp	Crayfish
Beef liver	Chicken liver
Organ meats	Fish roe
Sardines	Oysters
Vegetables	
Dried beans and peas	Baked beans
Black beans	Lentils
Chick peas	Lima beans
Kidney beans	Split peas
Northern beans	Soybeans

Other foods	
Bran cereals	Brewer's yeast
Nuts	Caramels
Whole grain products	Wheat germ
Seeds	

What to do if your phosphorus is too high? If your phosphorus is too high, consider what you are eating in your diet and substitute lower phosphorous foods. Talk to your dietitian about making changes in your diet, or your physician about a phosphate binder for you to take with meals.

Sodium

Healthy kidneys control how much sodium is in your body. If your kidneys are not functioning well, excess sodium causes fluid buildup, swelling and causes high blood pressure and strain on your heart. Your dietician or physician will advise the correct amount of sodium you should consume daily.

Instead of using salt, or salt substitutes which contain high levels of phosphorous, try using fresh garlic, fresh onion, garlic powder, onion powder, black pepper, lemon juice, vinegar and olive oil.

Maintaining a healthy weight and following a balanced meal plan that is low in salt can help you control your blood pressure. If you have diabetes, your meal plan is also important in controlling your blood sugar. Controlling high blood pressure and diabetes may also help slow down kidney disease.

According to the National Kidney Foundation, the following are the guidelines and reasons to follow a low protein diet if you have CKD.

Protein is necessary for growth as well as upkeep and repair of all parts of your body. Protein comes from the food you eat. When you digest it, the waste product of protein is called urea. If the kidneys are not working properly, urea builds up in the bloodstream, and can cause loss of appetite and fatigue. If you eat a low protein diet, the workload of the kidneys is reduced to preserve the health of the kidney that is still functioning.[10]

It is important to eat some of each type of protein daily. The two primary sources of protein are:

1. Animal protein considered high-quality proteins: fish, poultry, meat, eggs and dairy products. Dairy products needs to be limited because they are high in phosphorous.

2. Vegetable proteins considered low-quality proteins: bread, pasta, cereals, rice and dried beans.

How to stretch the protein you eat

You can stretch a small amount of protein so that it becomes more satisfying, by increasing the amount of vegetables, combined with rice or pasta. See the lists of low phosphorous, low potassium foods. Examples of recipes may be found in chapter 10.

---

10   NKF, 2015 https://www.kidney.org/atoz/content/sodiumckd,

Main Dishes

- Think of vegetables as the main dish, and meat as the side dish that complements the meal.

- Try making kebabs, using smaller pieces of meat and more vegetables

- Make rice or pasta, using more vegetables and less meat.

- Make a chef's salad using crisp vegetables and small strips of meat or egg.

- If you are making casseroles, decrease the amount of meat, and increase the amount of carbohydrate, low phosphorous and low potassium vegetables like carrots and celery.

- Use low sodium soups, when a recipe calls for it

- Use stronger tasting cheese, like cheddar or parmesan, as you will need less of it, for the same amount of flavor.

- When making sandwiches, use minimal protein and fill with lettuce, cucumber, chopped celery, apple, parsley or water chestnuts.

- Use lower protein foods, such as milk substitutes in soups, or rice and pasta, to make soups more robust without using too much protein.

Calorie Boosters

When you decrease the amount of protein, you are also reducing the number of calories in your diet. Maintaining a healthy weight is important. To make up for the loss of calories, try:

- use olive oil or other kidney healthy fats

- Increase healthy sweeteners: organic sugar, honey, stevia, jam and jello

The suggested diet is complex and needs to be under the supervision of an expert. I highly recommend working with someone to guide you with menu planning in order to ensure you are getting sufficient macro- and micro-nutrients, as well as calories. Staying as healthy as possible is essential, as dialysis is extremely stressful on the body.

When having dialysis, it always amazed me to see people eating salty, high fat foods, such as French fries, and drinking coca cola. It seemed so counterproductive to eat and drink food that would make you feel worse and not better. I encourage anyone on dialysis to follow the diet as closely as possible to help you move forward to a healthier and happier life. After all, "your health is your wealth."

Chapter 7

Transplanted

Our search for a kidney became the focal point of our lives. Steve was relentless in his pursuit of a match for me. He wrestled with all the intricate details and red tape involved in dealing with the various hospitals to get me registered on several transplant clinics' waiting lists. We were already listed at Emory Hospital and at the University of Minnesota Hospital for a cadaver kidney. The wait seemed interminably long, and we decided to pursue other avenues for me to have the transplant sooner rather than later.

We traveled to Louisville, Kentucky to register at the Jewish Hospital transplant unit there, having heard they received many type A blood kidney donors. After the lymphoma diagnosis, they refused to put me back on their transplant list until three years post treatment, by which time I would most likely not survive, or would be too weak to have transplant surgery.

We also traveled to the University of Alabama Hospital to register with their transplant unit.

Each hospital visit required an overnight hospital stay, while all the necessary tests were completed and I had to undergo my regular dialysis treatment. Each hospital visit, while emotionally draining and exhausting, was simultaneously charged with hope and possibility.

Steve left no stone unturned. He became my health advocate and my voice when I was too weak to speak. We registered in Alabama for the regular kidney transplant cadaver list as well as the paired donation list. This was an emerging trend for people waiting for a kidney transplant, providing they had someone willing to donate a kidney on their behalf who was not a match for them. They would have to be willing to pay it forward for someone else.

The Alliance for Paired Donation was founded by Mike Rees, MD, a transplant surgeon at the University of Toledo Medical Center. It is a non-profit organization designed for people who need a kidney transplant, and have a family member or friend who is not a match, willing to donate. The names, blood types, tissue types, and all other relevant information is entered into a database of patient-and-donor pairs, and the computer matches would be donors and recipients.[11]

The system is reliant on an honor system. Once the sick patient has been transplanted, the friend or family member needs to honor their promise. Having watched loved ones suffer for so long, no one has ever reneged on their promise.

---

11   Lorenzo Benet, The Kidney Cha. People Magazine Article Nov 30, 2009, pg70

The donor undergoes x-rays, scans, multiple blood draws, and psychological evaluations to deem them sufficiently mentally and physically healthy. Only then do they get the go-ahead to donate. The recipient is then able to get a living kidney donor, which generally speaking, lasts twice long as a cadaver kidney. Best of all, the process of being transplanted happens much sooner. This is a blessing for patients and their families who are anxiously waiting for years on end for an appropriate cadaver match.

Our last resort was to register at Johns Hopkins Hospital in Baltimore as participants in this paired donation program. In December 2007, Steve and I made our final attempt at registering at a hospital and registered with the incompatible kidney transplant team at Johns Hopkins, in a desperate attempt to find a suitable kidney for me. By January 2008, we were already being considered as part of a chain of 20 donors and recipients spanning the country, from Phoenix, Arizona, where the first transplant was to be performed, to Baltimore, Maryland where Steve and I ultimately had our surgeries.

On February 28, 2008, I received my last dialysis treatment. Gaby flew in from college and my dear friend Debbie joined us in loving support of the three of us. The morning before the surgery, my surgeon, Robert Montgomery, MD arrived in my hospital room and sat down as if for a friendly chat.

"I have good news and bad news," he said casually, as

he stroked his signature mustache. Breathless in antici-pation, I asked for the bad news first.

"It turns out they have not done the final cross-match, which is necessary before the kidney is trans-planted, he said. "Although it is simply a formality and most likely a non-issue."

Cross matching is used by doctors to make sure that the specific donor blood does not react with the patient's blood. It is basically a transfusion done in a test tube. The process takes 45 minutes to an hour and should have been done at least three days prior to the transplant.

"What does that mean for me?" I asked anxiously. Having said farewell to dialysis the previous day, I was unprepared and unwilling to resume the agonizing treatments once again.

"Well, you have two choices, and that is the good news," he said with a smile. "Steve is in the operating room right now as we speak. We can therefore either: a) Halt the nephrectomy until the cross-match is com-plete and proceed with your transplant, thereafter; or b) We can go ahead and remove Steve's kidney now, and proceed with your transplant after the cross-match is completed."

The severity of the situation hung over us like a dark cloud. However, Debbie quickly exclaimed, "If Steve wakes up after surgery and is told that he donated his kidney, but Janice has not yet been transplanted, he will be devastated. His nephrectomy needs to be halted right now, for however long it takes. Once you are able to proceed with the transplant, you can go ahead with the nephrectomy."

I was given a Xanax to calm me down and Gaby, Debbie and I, simultaneously drifted into exhausted naps. By the time we woke up they were ready to wheel me into the operating room with the cross-match completed, without any antibody reaction and Steve's nephrectomy underway. His kidney was then airlifted to Wake Forest Medical School where his recipient was prepped and already awaiting its arrival.

As soon as the kidney was securely transplanted in my body, I started excreting urine at a rapid rate. The transplant was successful. The match was perfect. For my body, with so many pre-existing antibodies, this in itself was a miracle.

The high antibody levels were from pregnancy and from the first double organ transplant. I also had several blood transfusions while on treatment for the lymphoma, due to a low white cells blood count and hemoglobin level. These transfusions escalated the already high antibody level.

The surgery proved to be extremely complicated, which made my transplant surgeon the ideal choice to perform the surgery. With so much scar tissue from previous surgeries, Dr. Montgomery needed to peel back layers upon layers of scar tissue before proceeding. In his own words, Dr. Montgomery has said, "Transplantation is dramatic. You take a person who's extremely ill and in many cases someone who is going to die, in some cases very soon, and you put a healthy organ into them and it just transforms them."

He said he particularly likes the challenge of transplanting organs in complex cases such as mine, and getting to know the patients and their families.

The day after surgery, I already felt remarkably well and began eating a normal diet. However, Steve did not fare as well as I did. After making a small incision in Steve's abdomen to remove his kidney laparoscopically, the doctors realized they had to abandon that approach and remove his kidney the old fashioned way with a much larger incision in the lower abdomen. Steve's pain level was extraordinary compared to mine. I was ready to be discharged from the hospital after four days but Steve was in no shape or form to leave for several more days, and then had to be readmitted.

I felt revived after a short time. However Steve's vulnerability and extreme pain made me ponder whether we had made the right decision. I wondered how much longer I could have held on while having hemodialysis. I wonder now if I would be writing this book today, had we waited for a cadaver kidney?

We remained in Baltimore nearby the hospital for a month post-surgery, so we could do lab work daily, have the surgeons monitor our progress carefully, and reverse any symptoms of rejection should they occur.

Steve's sense of humor prevailed despite his terrible pain. He joked about withdrawing his donation, and how he had given me his hand in marriage, his heart, and now his kidney.

We returned to Atlanta, with me walking off the plane. I had arrived in Baltimore in a wheelchair just four weeks prior.

After returning home, life seemed to settle down. Steve's health reinvigorated slowly but surely, and with that, my guilt at having been the reason for his pain dissipated.

It took me a long time to accept and believe that I was now able to live my life without worrying about dialysis treatments. I slowly began to accept and trust that I was a mother full of energy and radiant wellbeing. Finally, we were able to conduct our lives in healthy optimism, rather than uncertainty and anguish.

Through Steve's donation, he directly changed the lives of two people, and indirectly of so many more. He changed the trajectory of our family's future from one of despair and fear to one of hope and happiness.

After we arrived home from Baltimore, my sister Bonita came from Melbourne to nurse us back to health. Bonita had always been my very own Florence Nightingale. After every surgery and health crisis she would put her busy life on hold and come to our aid, ready to help in any way she could. With her loving and gentle encouragement, we were both able to recover and thrive.

I gained strength both physically and emotionally, and celebrated my fiftieth birthday a few days after we arrived home, in good health and spirits, surrounded by my loving family. My gift, a family vacation in Bermuda. The first vacation in four years.

Chapter 8

Eating My Way to Recovery and Radiant Health

"I don't need fillers, additives, excess amounts of sugars,
fats, salts and other measures taken to taint
the natural goodness of real food"
Dr. Mark Hyman MD[12]

While I was on dialysis and having Retuxin treatments, a friend from New Jersey came to visit. Her mother had been battling cancer for several years and she opened my eyes to the concept that eating an organic diet was not an expensive fad, but an essential part of healing and thriving. This was later reinforced while studying at the Institute of Integrative Nutrition®.

I began to understand that one cannot fuel his/her body and achieve optimal health if he/she eats food packed with toxic chemicals and genetically modified organisms.

---

12   Dr. Mark Hymen "Quotes by Mark Hyman." @ Like Success. N.p.,n.d. Web. 06 Apr. 2016

Originally, all food was grown organically and was eaten unrefined in its original form with minimal processing. However, since World War 2, there has been a rise in chemical farming and food processing. The soil and the food in many parts of the world have been depleted of essential minerals and nutrients. Pesticides and herbicides create additional work for the immune system, often resulting in diseases, such as cancer, liver, kidney and blood diseases.

Eating organically helps you to reduce the toxic burden in your body's immune system and cleanse your body of toxic build up. It is important to check labels and make sure that 100 percent USDA Certified Organic is on the label, or you may risk eating non-organic ingredients. This organic certification is the best assurance that the produce you are eating has been grown and handled according to strict guidelines.

The best way to eat an organic diet is to eat whole, seasonal, unprocessed (or minimally processed), organic food. Organic produce is by definition non GMO and includes both plants and animals, which have not been treated with pesticides, herbicides, fertilizers, radiation, growth hormones or antibiotics.

Most conventionally raised animals are fed with a combination of soy and corn, of which 90 percent is genetically modified. The food is packed with hormones and antibiotics, as well as bovine growth hormone in dairy cows to increase lactation. The antibiotics given to animals prevent infections, but also make their way along with hormones, into our dairy produce and into our bodies.

GMOs comprise a large percentage of commercial soy, corn, alfalfa, and beets in the United States. They change crops in order to make them weather and pest resistant. The pest-resistant Btoxin used for this purpose not only kills pests, but also pokes holes in human beings, damaging the intestines and causing leaky gut syndrome. These toxins are in the DNA of the produce and cannot be washed off, contrary to popular belief.

Immediately after my transplant, I began to enjoy all the foods that I had been denied for so long while I was on dialysis. Part of a successful recovery is good nutrition. After any surgery, adequate protein and calories are essential for proper wound healing as well as overcoming the muscle breakdown caused by high doses of prednisone. I had lost so much muscle tissue and had become so emaciated over the course of two years on dialysis, that adequate protein was an essential component to my healing process.

The best types of protein post-transplantation are lean cuts of beef, skinless poultry, wild caught fish (mostly salmon), eggs (limited to three or four yolks per week) and low fat dairy.

Nuts and legumes are also good sources of protein for vegetarians. Soy protein should always be organic, due to the widespread genetically modified soy bean crops.

Concentrated carbohydrates need to be limited, as steroid medications tend to elevate blood sugar levels.

It is important to read labels carefully to make sure you are not taking in any unwanted, hidden sugars in the form of honey, sucrose, dextrose, fructose or corn syrup. Eating unrefined, whole unprocessed carbohydrate is always going to be the best option.

Prednisone can also increase sodium and water retention, as well as blood pressure. Therefore, sodium needs to be restricted. The no-salt diet is best. Salt substitutes often contain high levels of potassium and should be used with caution. I generally find that the natural taste of local, seasonal, fresh organic fruit and vegetables to be so delicious that I do not need salt at all.

Potassium is increased with certain immune suppressant drugs, such as Prograf or Cyclosporin. When potassium concentration is too high, it can cause heart problems with muscle cramping. It is advisable to check serum potassium levels and adapt your diet accordingly.

A heart healthy diet is highly recommended, where you are avoiding high saturated fat foods and increasing the amount of fiber in your diet. A high-fiber diet may also help to lower cholesterol. Always strive to choose whole grains over refined grains and to eat more fresh fruit and a combination of raw and cooked vegetables.

It is recommended to avoid eating grapefruit or drinking any grapefruit juice as it interferes with certain medications. You should also avoid raw fish or meat, such as sushi or oysters. Raw or undercooked eggs are also not recommended, as is unpasteurized milk or dairy. Cheese with mold, such as blue cheese or stilton should also be avoided as you may be at higher risk for getting sick from the mold. After the restricted diet I followed while on dialysis, I could happily live with these restrictions.

It is easy to gain weight after a transplant, due to the medications, as well as the freedom to enjoy the food you had previously been restricted from eating. This can lead to type 2 diabetes, as well as to heart issues and needs to be monitored carefully. I recommend working with a health coach like me, who is well versed in post-transplant diets, to help you implement both diet and lifestyles changes and avoid unnecessary weight gain.

Exercise should also become part of your daily regimen. It should last for at least 30 to 40 minutes per session. Self-care in the form of meditation and yoga are great ways to relax and calm your mind and your body.

It is also vital to get adequate sleep. I frequently utilize Andrew Weil, MD's method of relaxing and calming my mind, by incorporating the four, seven, eight breathing program into my nightly routine. First, I relax my body and breathe in for four seconds, hold it for seven, and then slowly breathe out for eight seconds. I repeat this several times, until I fall asleep. It is wonderful how easily you can get into a meditative, relaxed state by implementing this simple technique.

Once my incision had adequately healed, I was finally able to get back to Pilates, take a spin class and go walking-- all of which I had sorely missed doing.

Steve and I would take our beloved Labrador retrievers George and Charlie for long walks around our neighborhood. I never took for granted the fact that I had not been able to participate in this activity just a short while previously.

I also began to experiment with cooking, using different spices and ingredients. I found new chefs to follow Including Yottam Ottolenghi, Sharon Glass and Levana Kirschenbaum, just to name a few. I poured over their cookbooks, eager to try out different recipes and translate them into healthier versions for my family to enjoy.

I had finally found my true calling and passion. Cooking became not just an essential part of my everyday life, but also a way of coping and healing. It was also my way of translating everything that had transpired into something positive, creative and delectable.

Part 2

Recipes

Don't eat anything your great-grandmother wouldn't recognize as food."[13]
Michael Pollan

---

13   Pollan, Michael. *Food Rules: An Eater's Manual.* New York: Penguin, 2009.
Print.

Chapter 9

Diabetic Friendly and Low GI Recipes

My "entrée" into the world of cooking began after taking cooking lessons in Johannesburg with my sister, Bonita and my mother. We would gather in the evenings once a week, sit and watch the magic unfold, and then go home and try the recipes out for ourselves.

Bonita and I have traded recipes back and forth across the miles for years. Now Gaby is an active participant in our recipe swap.

I am grateful to Sybil Smerkowitz, June Edelmuth, and Myrna Rosen, as well as to my mother, for inspiring me to express myself creatively through the art of cooking. I grew up watching, tasting, smelling, sharing and experiencing life in my mother's well-used kitchen. Food and cooking were catalysts for discussion, and expressions of love and celebration.

The following are some recipes that sustained me as a type 1 diabetic during childhood, adolescence and young adulthood. I have adapted several recipes to be diabetic friendly as well as to remain faithful to my philosophy of eating real, clean and whole food.

Monkey Gland Steak

This is a traditional sauce served with steak. It is spicy and delicious.

Serves 4

Ingredients and Directions

4 Grass fed, organic skirt steaks. Season with salt and pepper. Grill in a pan or on an open grill, until desired preference. Keep warm.

Chop 2 onions and fry in olive oil till golden brown. Add 2 large skinned and diced tomatoes and cook for 8 -10 minutes. Add 1 chicken cube, 1 cup of water, 1 cup organic ketchup, ½ cup Worcester sauce, 1 TB soy sauce, ½ cup hot chutney, 1 tsp brown sugar or honey, and salt and pepper to taste. Simmer until boiling, and pour over steak and serve. Sprinkle chopped parsley over for garnish.

~~~~~~~~~~~~~~~~~~~~~~~~~~~~~~~~~~~~~~~

Chicken Soup

The "Jewish Penicillin," and number one comfort food in every household. Holidays and sick days alike would never be quite the same without a pot of this healing broth simmering on the stove top, and without the distinctive aroma permeating the entire house. The vegetables and chicken in the soup make for a complete, low-GI meal. Serve with a green salad.

Serves 6-8

Ingredients
1 beef shank bone
1 whole organic chicken, fat trimmed
6 carrots thinly sliced
1 onion quartered and studded with 4 cloves
2/3 sticks of celery thinly sliced
1 cup of cubed butternut squash
Handful of parsley coarsely chopped
Handful of fresh dill coarsely chopped
2 turnips peeled and chopped
2-3 parsnips peeled and chopped
2-3 leeks, white part only, washed and thinly chopped
3 teaspoons kosher salt
Few dashes of white pepper to taste
4 chicken bouillon cubes

Directions
Wash and soak meat in 1 TB of salt and boiling water for 15-20 minutes. While meat is soaking, fill a large stock pot ¾ full of water and bring to the boil. Add meat and vegetables, and allow it to simmer gently for 5-6 hours. Skim fat off the top periodically. Add seasonings, parsley, and dill, and remove meat. You can remove the skin and bones of the chicken and cut into bite-size pieces and put back into to the soup, or use separately. Adjust seasonings according to personal taste. I like to leave the vegetables in the broth, or you can strain the liquid and discard the cooked vegetables. You can also add noodles if desired and simmer until noodles are cooked for about 10-15 minutes.

Our Family Favorite Roast Chicken

Nothing is quite as satisfying as a roast chicken. The pleasant aroma during the cooking process pervades the entire house and alludes to a delicious and sumptuous feast.

This recipe adapted from Jamie Oliver is one of our family favorites. Begin by patting the skin dry, and trimming off the excess fat. Carefully separate the skin on top of the breast, and the back and stuff with an array of fresh chopped herbs. Fill the cavity with 2 bay leaves, a lemon cut in half, fresh sprigs of rosemary and thyme herbs, 1 or 2 garlic cloves and an onion cut in half.

Serves 6

Ingredients

One 2-3 lb free range organic chicken
Kosher salt and fresh pepper
3 handfuls fresh herbs. I use parsley, rosemary, sage, thyme and basil.
2-3 TB olive oil
I lemon cut in half
2-3 bay leaves
2 cloves garlic

Directions

Preheat the oven to 425 degrees F. Wash chicken inside and out and pat dry. Rub cavity with salt and pepper. Gently pull the skin away from the breast, thigh and drumstick, and fill with finely chopped herbs, moving hands gently towards the middle. After the legs have been tied together, and herbs are pushed under the skin, rub salt and pepper all over the chicken, as well as the remaining herbs. Tuck the winglets under and pull the skin of the breast forward so that the flesh is not exposed. Rub with olive oil, place in a roasting pan, and roast for 1 ½ to 2 hours, until fragrant and crispy. Serve with roasted potatoes and green salad.

~~~~~~~~~~~~~~~~~~~~~~~~~~~~~~~~~~~~~~~

Quick Roast Chicken with Balsamic Vinegar and Rosemary or Thyme

This is adapted from a Sharon Glass recipe, from her book "Absolutely Delicious".

When time is of the essence but you are in the mood for a delicious and gratifying homemade roast chicken, this recipe always comes to mind. It can be marinated overnight, or for just a few hours before cooking, and is always a hit in our home. It is wonderfully simple and delicious.

Serves 6

Ingredients
1 2-3 lb. free range chicken
3 TB fresh or 2 TB dried rosemary or thyme
½ cup balsamic vinegar
1 tsp crushed garlic
2 TB olive oil
Kosher salt and pepper.

Directions

Spatchcock the chicken, by cutting down the breast bone, and flattening open with your hands. Turn so skin faces up. Make a marinade with the oil, vinegar herbs, and garlic. Season both sides with salt and pepper, and pour marinade over both sides.

Preheat oven to 400 degrees F, and cook for 1 ½ hours, turning half way and basting frequently, until brown and crisp.

~~~~~~~~~~~~~~~~~~~~~~~~~~~~~~~~~~~~~

Heirloom Tomato Salad

This salad, adapted from Sharon Glass, is my favorite summer salad. It makes a beautiful presentation. Use whichever tomatoes are in season to enhance the taste. The dressing can be made a few days ahead and stored in the refrigerator.

Serves 6

Ingredients

3 ½ oz. multi colored cherry tomatoes
3 ½ oz. mini Rosa tomatoes or grape tomatoes
3 ½ oz. organic heirloom tomatoes, multi colored
¾ organic Roma tomatoes
Handful of fresh basil leaves
2 mini cucumbers, sliced thinly
½ red onion, peeled and thinly sliced
½ avocados
2 to 3 cups mixed baby lettuces, washed and dried thoroughly

Directions
Wash and dry all tomatoes thoroughly and cut into different shapes and sizes. Place lettuces, cucumbers, and onions in a salad bowl, Wash and dry the basil and tear into small pieces and place in the bowl along with the tomatoes. Cut avocado into chunks and place in the bowl. Dress about ½ an hour before serving.

Dressing
½ cup olive oil
¼ cup fresh squeezed lemon juice
1 tsp dry mustard
1 tsp honey
Coarse salt and pepper to taste

Directions
Whisk all ingredients together and pour over salad just before serving. I use this dressing for mixed green salads as well.

Additional diabetic friendly recipes in chapters 10, 11, 12 , 13, 14 and 15.

Chapter 10

Recipes for a Diet Low in Protein, Phosphorous, Potassium and Sodium

The following recipes are some examples of dishes I made while I did not have a healthy functioning kidney. These recipes are great choices when reducing protein quantities, by adding in low potassium vegetables and spices.

~~~~~~~~~~~~~~~~~~~~~~~~~~~

Chicken and Vegetable Risotto

This recipe is an example of using minimal protein, and stretching it into a satisfying and delicious meal. I love making this dish, even when not reducing protein, phosphorous and potassium.

Serves 8

Ingredients
4 Organic free range chicken breasts cut into strips
¼ cup olive oil
1 onion chopped
1 tsp garlic crushed
3 large carrots chopped
2 cups Arborio Italian rice
1 cup white wine
2 ½ cups low sodium chicken stock
½ cup dried porcini mushrooms
2 tomatoes diced
6 zucchini chopped in ½ inch pieces
½ cup frozen petit peas
½ cup organic corn kernels, rinse if using canned or use sodium free
2 TB chopped parsley
1 tsp dry sage
Pepper and sodium free seasoning

Directions
Soak porcini mushrooms in ¾ cup boiling water for about 10 minutes. Preheat oven to 400 degrees F.

Sauté chicken in 2 TB olive oil till seared and half cooked. Set aside. In the same pan, sauté onion, garlic and carrots in remaining oil until golden.

Add dry uncooked rice, sauté for a few minutes, stirring constantly.

Mix white wine, chicken stock and liquid from mushrooms together and pour 1 ½ cups slowly over rice, stirring constantly to ensure it is absorbed. After a few minutes, add porcini mushrooms, zucchini, and corn. Pour remaining liquid over rice and vegetables, stir in parsley, sage, and lots of seasonings. Toss in the ½ cooked chicken.

Place everything into an ovenproof casserole with a fitted lid, and bake for 25 minutes, or until rice is soft and almost all the liquid is absorbed. Stir in tomatoes and petit peas and serve immediately.

~~~~~~~~~~~~~~~~~~~~~~~~~~~~~~~~~~~

Turkey Meatloaf My Way

This is another example of minimizing the amount of protein, by substituting with vegetables. We love this dish! It is immensely satisfying and delicious.

Serves 6

Ingredients
1 TB olive oil
1 chopped onion
1 stick chopped celery
6 chopped brown mushrooms
2 cloves garlic
1 scallion chopped
1 tsp thyme
1 TB parsley
¼ cup chopped tomato
1 TB balsamic vinegar

Dash chili flakes
½ cup gluten-free breadcrumbs
1 beaten egg
½ lb. organic ground turkey breast
1 onion sliced

Directions

Preheat oven to 375 degrees F.

Heat oil and sauté onion, celery, mushrooms, garlic, scallion and thyme, for about 6-8 minutes and season with no salt seasoning and pepper. Allow to cool, and transfer to a bowl. In a separate bowl add parsley, tomatoes, vinegar, and chili. Add egg slightly beaten, breadcrumbs, and then turkey. Mix in the vegetable mixture and mix well.

Transfer to an oiled baking pan, and shape in a loaf. Slice an onion and place over loaf, and then drizzle remaining olive oil. Cover with foil and bake for an hour. Uncover and spoon over the pan juices, then return to the oven for another half an hour, spooning over juices every 10/15 minutes. Enjoy with a green salad on the side.

If not reducing potassium, I slice several thick slices of tomato and a potato and place it on top of the onion, before drizzling with olive oil and baking.

Lamb or Beef Casserole

Adapted from Sharon Glass's book, "Absolutely Delicious."

Serves 8-10

Ingredients

2 lbs. beef or lamb cut into medium size chunks
Pepper and 1 tsp salt
3 TB olive oil
2 large carrots, chopped
1 onion chopped
3 sticks celery, chopped
2 cups dry red wine
1 TB juniper berries
2 tsp chopped garlic
2 sprigs rosemary
3 cups water

Directions

Season meat with lots of black pepper and 1 tsp salt, or salt substitute and brown in batches in olive oil. Set aside and pour off excess oil.

Place all ingredients, except water, in a large casserole and simmer on low heat for approximately two hours, stirring every half an hour. Add 1 cup of water at a time, if necessary, so the meat does not dry out, and it makes a delicious sauce.

This is best made a day or two ahead, so the meat becomes soft and tender, and the entire dish develops a unique taste.

~~~~~~~~~~~~~~~~~~~~~~~~~~~~~~~~~~~~~

Chicken Satay with Basmati Rice
Serves 6

This is another gratifying and delicious dish, adapted from Sharon Glass, with a combination of the rice, chicken and vegetables. The rice is made first as it takes the longest.

Ingredients

Spiced Basmati Rice
1 tsp coriander seeds
1 tsp mustard seeds
2 tsp olive oil
1 ½ cups basmati white rice
1 ¾ cups low sodium chicken stock
1 bay leaf
1 tsp paprika

Heat coriander and mustard seeds in a medium size pot, on high, until they begin to pop. Add dry rice and sauté for a few minutes. Remove from the stove, add hot chicken stock, bay leaf and paprika. Wait 5 minutes for the rice to soften, then place back on the stove for about 15-20 minutes, until all liquid has evaporated and rice is fluffy. Set aside.

Satay Sauce
1-2 TB low sodium soy sauce
1-2 TB mirin
1 tsp fresh ginger
1 tsp chopped garlic
1 TB lime juice
Pepper to taste
3 organic chicken breasts

Directions
Whisk all sauce ingredients together and set aside.

Make 2 slashes on top of each chicken breast, season with pepper and low salt seasoning. Brush with olive oil, and heat a grill or broiler. Once hot, sear chicken on either side until almost cooked. Place fillets in an ovenproof dish, and brush with half the satay sauce, and set aside. To reheat, grill directly under the grill for a few minutes.

Vegetables
10 oz. mixed broccoli, asparagus, white mushrooms, cauliflower and onion, cut up
1½ oz. carrots julienned
2 TB olive oil
Remainder of satay sauce

Directions
Stir fry the vegetables in a wok for 8-10 minutes on high. Add sauce and simmer until sauce thickens.

Place a portion of rice on each plate, followed by the vegetables and topped with half a chicken breast.

Horseradish Salmon
Serves 4

Gaby found this recipe in "Food and Wine" many years ago and it is a staple, not only in our kitchen, but in my sister's as well as all my nieces' kitchens in Australia. It is so simple and tasty, and there is no need for any salt. The horseradish contains little to no sodium, and this makes it a perfect recipe while you are on a sodium restricted diet. Make sure to choose wild caught salmon, and not farm raised Atlantic salmon.

Brush the glaze on the salmon in the last minute of grilling, so the sugars don't burn.

Ingredients
¼ cup plus 2 TB dijon mustard
¼ cup prepared horseradish, drained (I use white, but red is okay too)
2 TB honey
Four 6 oz. pieces of salmon fillet, skinless
Olive oil
Black pepper
Low sodium soy sauce or Coconut Aminos

Directions
Light a grill. In a small bowl, mix horseradish and honey. Rub the salmon with the oil, pepper, and salt (if not reducing sodium). Grill salmon over moderate heat, right side up, until lightly browned, about 3 minutes. Turn and grill 3 minutes longer, until the salmon is

almost cooked through. Turn again, and spread each fillet with 1 TB of the glaze. Turn and grill until well glazed, about 30 seconds.

May be served over a salad or with a side of vegetables and white rice.

~~~~~~

Roasted Cauliflower and Shallots

Adapted from Laura Zinn Fromm's book, "Sweet Survival"
Serves 6

Ingredients
1 large cauliflower
1 shallot thinly sliced
2-3 TB cup extra virgin olive oil
Zest and juice from 1 lemon
1-2 tsp no salt seasoning
1 tsp ground black pepper

Directions
Preheat oven to 425 degrees F.

Cut cauliflower into small flowerets, and spread on a baking tray along with the shallots. Drizzle olive oil, then sprinkle seasonings over the cauliflower. Pour lemon juice over, and then sprinkle zest.

Roast for 30 minutes until nice and brown and fragrant.

Put under broiler for 10-15 minutes to brown further.

Moroccan Carrot Salad

This salad makes an attractive addition to the dinner table. It is adapted from Sharon Glass, and is another family favorite. It makes for a tasty low GI carbohydrate alternative.

Serves 4

Ingredients
1 lb. baby carrots, with stems

Vinaigrette
½ cup olive oil
¼ cup red wine vinegar
1 TB lemon
1 TB sweet paprika
½ tsp minced garlic
¼ cup chopped parsley
Fresh mint leaves for garnish
Coarse salt and pepper to taste

Boil carrots until tender but firm. Drain, cool and set aside.

Whisk all ingredients for the dressing together and pour over the carrots. Leave at room temperature to marinade, top with slivers of chopped mint and serve.

Baked Apples
Serves 6

Ingredients
6 apples, such as Golden Delicious, Rome or
Macintosh
½ cup organic brown sugar
4 TB unsalted grass fed butter
½ cup water
1-2 tsp ground cinnamon
½ tsp lemon zest
4 TB peach preserves

Directions
Preheat oven to 375 degrees F.

Core the apples cutting to within 1" of the base, leaving
base intact. Combine ½ of sugar, 2 TB butter, water, 1/4
tsp cinnamon and lemon zest and bring to a boil. Mix
preserves with remaining butter, sugar and cinnamon
and fill the apples with mixture. Arrange apples in a
baking dish, pour over brown sugar syrup and bake
until easily pierced and brown. Pour over juice from the
pan regularly. Slip under the broiler for a few minutes
to brown further.

Enjoy with a scoop of low potassium fruit sorbet or
sherbet.

Our Family's Favorite Apple Caramel Cake
Serves 8-10

Ingredients
3 TB butter
1 cup organic sugar
Cream together, and then add 3 eggs, one at a time,
while mixing
1 cup flour
1 tsp baking powder
Pinch of salt
½ cup rice milk

Add all ingredients to egg mixture, and mix well.

Place in a large pie dish.

Arrange slices of 2 peeled and cored apples or 1 large
can pie apples.

Bake at 375 degrees F for 45 minutes

Sauce
1 cup nondairy cream such as Riches
1 cup sugar
1 tsp vanilla essence
Bring all ingredients to a boil.

Once the cake is out the oven, pierce with a fork, and
spoon over sauce immediately.

Chapter 11

Soup, My Ultimate Comfort Food

After my second transplant, I was determined to eat healthfully, while still satisfying my food cravings. Comfort food means different things to different people. To Steve, comfort food is a hearty stew or a fragrant curry. To me, it's the intoxicating warmth and allure of a steaming bowl of soup. Nothing quite beats the comfort, or is quite as healing and satisfying to me than a steaming bowl of broth.

Dating back to my mother's chicken soup, which infused every nook and cranny of the house with its transformative aroma, I have always craved the comfort of soup. On a cold winter's day, its seductive warmth draws me. In summertime, its cooling properties help combat the heat.

Either way, hearty or light, chunky or smooth, hot or cold soup, using seasonal, local ingredients is a great way to nourish yourself and your family. It is a nutritionally dense and relatively low cost dish. Furthermore, what I love most about soup is the bonding ritual of sitting down together and eating.

These are some of my favorite recipes.

Roasted Red Pepper and Tomato Soup

Sharon Glass's recipe, from her book, "Simply Too Delicious," is a great hit every time I make it. The roasting of the vegetables brings out the umami and the sweetness. Tomatoes, once cooked, also have that deeply satisfying umami quality, or fifth taste. According to Micheal Polan, author of *Cooked, a Natural History*, "Umami is the quasi secret heart and soul of every braise, stew and soup."[14]

We love the spicy kick, but if you don't care for it, leave it out.

Serves 6-8

Ingredients

3 large red peppers
1 onion
3 large carrots
2 sticks celery
¼ cup olive oil
½ tsp. chili paste
14 oz. can crushed tomatoes

---

14   Pollan, Michel. *Cooked , a Natural History*. N.p.: n.p., n.d. Web.

5 sun dried tomatoes in vinaigrette
1/3 cup vinaigrette from sun dried tomatoes
4 cups boiling water
4 TB vegetable or chicken stock
½ cup coconut milk (I use light coconut milk)
Coarse salt and pepper

Directions
Place peppers in a baking tray directly under the broiler and blacken all over. Allow to cool, and then peel skin. Remove seeds, chop and set aside. You can do this several days in advance and store in an air tight container in the refrigerator.

Reheat oven to 400 degrees F.

Place onion, carrots and celery in a food processor, and chop coarsely. Place in a roasting pan, along with olive oil, chili paste, canned tomatoes, sun dried tomatoes, vinaigrette, salt and pepper. Roast for 30 minutes uncovered, then add the peppers, and roast another 15 minutes.

Cool and place in stock pot with the water, chicken stock, and use an immersion blender to blend till smooth. Add coconut milk and additional salt and pepper to taste. Heat and serve.

If you do not care for coconut milk, leave it out. You can make this soup 2 or 3 days ahead of time.

Roasted Butternut and Chickpea Soup

This recipe has been adapted from "Cooking with the Raizons 3". A book by sisters, Lana and Delia, in Melbourne, Australia. I love the combination of tasty, seasonal vegetables and spices. This soup makes a complete meal, as the chickpeas are a great source of protein.

Ingredients

1 medium butternut squash, peeled and cut into chunks
2 cloves garlic, crushed
1 Spanish onion, chopped in segments
1 golden delicious apple, peeled, cored and chopped
1 tsp. grated ginger
2 TB olive oil 2 tsp cumin
6 cups prepared chicken stock
2 cans 400 gm chickpeas, rinsed and drained
Salt and black pepper to taste

Directions:

Preheat oven to 400 degrees F.

Combine butternut squash, garlic, onion, apple and ginger in an ovenproof dish, toss with olive oil, coarse salt and pepper, and bake for 40 minutes. Transfer to a large pot and add stock, and one can of chickpeas. Bring to a boil, then reduce and cover, simmering for 30 minutes. Use an immersion blender to blend until smooth. Add remaining can of chickpeas and reheat. Season according to taste with additional salt and pepper.

Mushroom Soup

This recipe has been adapted from Sharon Glass' book, "Simply Delicious." Mushrooms are known for their rich flavor, and when cooked are transformed to contain umami, or that deeply satisfying fifth taste normally found only in animal products. Mushrooms are antioxidants and contain many essential vitamins and minerals. The creamy texture, enhanced by the rosemary and sherry, makes this soup rich and delicious.

Ingredients

2 TB olive oil 1 TB butter

1 onion, chopped

1 leek, sliced thinly

1 TB fresh rosemary

1 lb. medium brown mushrooms, sliced

8 oz. white mushrooms, sliced

¼ cup flour (I use gluten free)

3 cups chicken or vegetable stock

Salt and pepper

1 cup unsweetened almond milk, or regular milk

1 TB liquid Amino's (which are gluten free) or soy sauce

Pinch of sugar

2 TB sherry

Preparation

Heat oil and butter. Add onion and leeks and allow to soften. Do not brown.

Add rosemary and brown mushrooms, and fry until

softened. Add flour and cook for 1 minute, then add stock and allow to thicken. Season with salt and pepper, place lid on the pot and simmer for 15 minutes.

Puree with an immersion blender until smooth. Place back on stove and add remaining button mushrooms, milk, liquid aminos and sugar, and simmer for 10 minutes. I sometimes add a handful of dehydrated porcini mushrooms at this point to enhance the flavor even more, and bring out the umami. Stir in sherry, and serve.

May add chopped parsley for garnish.

~~~~~~

Moroccan Lentil Soup (Harira)

Levana Kirschenbaum's lentil soup from her book, "Levana's Table," has a rich and deeply satisfying flavor. The comforting meaty quality of the lentils is delicious. Turmeric, besides being delicious, has long been known for its healing, anti-inflammatory qualities, which makes this a highly nutritious soup.

Serves 12

Ingredients
2 cups green or brown lentils
6 cups water
2 large onions
1 large bunch flat leaf parsley
1 small bunch cilantro, tough end and stem cut off

6 ribs celery, peeled
4 cups canned crushed tomatoes
1/3 cup olive oil
2 tsp turmeric
Salt to taste
12 cups water
2 TB cumin
¼ cup fresh lemon juice
Fresh ground pepper to taste

Directions
In a food processor, finely grind the onion, parsley, cilantro and celery. Transfer the mixture to a heavy wide-bottom pot. Add all but the last ingredient and bring to the boil. Reduce the heat to medium and cook covered for 1 hour, or a little longer until the lentils are perfectly tender and the soup looks thick and creamy. Stir in the cumin, lemon juice and black pepper and cook another 5 minutes. Adjust the texture and seasonings and serve.

Variation
You can substitute the lentils with buckwheat, bulgur, teff, steel-cut oats or millet. These grains take only a few minutes to cook. Proceed with the recipe just as above, substituting 2 cups of the suggested grain for the lentils, but with one change. Add them in the last 20 minutes of cooking.

Serve hot.

Cold Pea and Basil Soup

This easy, refreshing and velvety soup adapted from Gwyneth Paltrow's book, "My Father's Daughter," is perfect for a hot summer's eve. You can also heat it up in winter, and is a favorite with children.

Ingredients
1 TB olive oil
1 large yellow onion, diced
4 cups frozen green peas
1 quart vegetable stock
12 large fresh organic basil leaves
Coarse salt and ground black pepper
Best quality olive oil for serving

Directions
Heat olive oil in a small soup pot over medium heat. Add onion and cook till soft, about 10 minutes.

Add peas and stock and bring to a boil. Reduce heat, cover and simmer for 10 minutes. Remove from the stove, add basil, salt and pepper to taste, and allow to cool. Use immersion blender to liquidize until smooth. Cool in refrigerator for at least 2 hours.

Serve garnished finely chopped basil and a dollop of olive oil.

Chapter 12

Meatless Mondays

Meatless Mondays have become a tradition in our household, and are even extended to a few extra meatless meals during the week.

Going meatless once a week may reduce your risk of chronic preventable conditions like cancer, cardiovascular disease, type 2 diabetes and obesity. It can also help reduce our carbon footprint and save precious resources like fossil fuels and fresh water.

Evidence suggests that eating a diet rich in fruits and vegetables, and a limited amount of red meat can increase longevity, whereas red and processed meat consumption can be associated with increases in deaths due to cancer and cardiovascular disease

Going meatless encourages consumption of plant-based sources of protein, like beans and peas. Consuming beans and peas results in a higher intake of fiber (which improves digestion), protein, folate, zinc, iron and magnesium.

Though it can be challenging to serve healthy meals

on a budget, going meatless once a week can help conserve money for more fruits and vegetables.

Why not make meatless Monday a tradition in your family meal plan?

Here are a few of our family favorites.

~~~~~~

Red Lentil Coconut Curry with Cauliflower
Adapted from Laura Zinn Fromm's book "Sweet Survival"

Serves 6-8

Ingredients
1 TB coconut oil
1 yellow onion, diced
3 cloves garlic, minced
1 tsp. cumin
1 TB medium curry spice
3 carrots, cut in ¼ inch pieces
Butternut squash or sweet potato, cut into ¼ inch pieces
1 cup red lentils
1 can coconut milk (I use light coconut milk)
1 cup chopped kale
Handful chopped cilantro
Sea salt and pepper to taste

Directions
In a large stockpot, heat coconut oil over medium heat. Sauté onion and garlic till soft. Add curry powder and cumin and stir to release flavors of the spices Add

carrots, cauliflower, sweet potato or butternut and stir, incorporating the curry into the vegetables. Rinse lentils thoroughly and add with vegetable broth. Turn heat to high, bring to a boil, then lower heat. Cover and simmer for 30 minutes, until veggies are soft and lentils are mushy. Remove from heat and add coconut milk, kale and cilantro. Season with salt and pepper.

Moroccan Chili with Harissa

I have adapted this recipe by Maggie Jones, from the online magazine, "One Green Planet," and have passed it along to my family members and clients, who all enjoy the rich combination of spices and textures, which give a unique twist to traditional chili.

Ingredients
1 tsp olive oil
1 medium yellow onion, diced
3 cloves garlic, minced
2 TB ras el-hanout
1 TB harissa
1 large sweet potato or 2 cups butternut, chopped in ¼ inch pieces
Two 15 oz. cans organic chickpeas, rinsed and drained
Two 15 oz. cans no salt added diced tomatoes
¼ cup tomato paste
¼ cup golden raisins
¼ cup cilantro, chopped

Ras El-Hanout Spice Blend
2 tsp ginger
2 tsp cardamom
2 tsp mace
2 tsp cinnamon
1 tsp allspice
1 tsp coriander
1 tsp nutmeg
1 tsp turmeric
1 tsp black pepper
½ tsp white pepper
½ tsp cayenne pepper
¼ tsp cloves

Directions

Heat oil in a heavy pot over medium heat. Add onions, garlic and sauté until softened, about 5 minutes. Add ras el-hanout and harissa and simmer another minute until fragrant. Stir in the tomatoes with juice, sweet potato and tomato paste. Cover and simmer, stirring occasionally, for about 30 minutes till soft. Stir in drained chickpeas and raisins. Simmer an additional 5 minutes until warmed through. Season to taste, adding more harissa for more heat. Top with cilantro and vegan feta, if desired. Serve hot.

Shakshuka

Serves 6

This traditional Israeli dish makes an amazing breakfast, lunch or dinner. You can omit the feta if you prefer.

Ingredients

¼ cup olive oil
1 cup chopped yellow onion
1 cup chopped green pepper
1 jalapeno, seeded and finely diced
4 cloves garlic, minced
1 quart canned chopped tomatoes
1 TB tomato paste
1 tsp paprika
6 eggs
1/3 heaped cup crumbled Israeli Feta cheese

Directions

In a large skillet, heat olive oil over medium heat, add onion, green pepper and jalapeno and cook till softened, about 7 minutes. Add garlic and cook another minute. Add chopped tomatoes, tomato paste and paprika and cook until thickened, about 15 minutes. Make 6 wells and crack an egg into each well. Cover pan and cook until desired doneness of the eggs. Remove from the heat and sprinkle with feta (if desired, or leave it out).

Chapter 13

Main Courses

For years we have been hearing about factory farming, and the cruel, punitive conditions that livestock are raised in. Whether appearing on a carton of eggs in your grocery store or listed on a menu in your favorite restaurant, words like "free-range," "grass-fed," "natural," and "organic" are printed on eggs, fish, poultry and beef alike.

New food label claims crop up regularly, so if you come across a new one, be sure to take some time to do your own research as to what it really means. These are a few of the most commonly used labels.

ANTIBIOTIC-FREE [15]

"Antibiotic-free" means that an animal was not given antibiotics during its lifetime. Other similar phrases include "no antibiotics administered" and "raised without antibiotics."

---

15   Institute of Integrative Nutrition® resources. © 2014, 2015 Integrative Nutrition Inc. IIN .

CAGE-FREE

"Cage-free" means that the poultry is not raised in cages. It does not explain whether they were pasture raised, if they had access to the outdoors, or if they were raised in overcrowded conditions indoors. When you are buying eggs, poultry or meat that was raised outdoors, make sure there is a label that says "pasture raised".

FREE-RANGE

The use of the term "free-range" is defined by the USDA for eggs and poultry production. The label can be used as long as the producers allow the poultry access to the outdoors so they are raised in a natural habitat. It does not necessarily mean that the products are cruelty free, antibiotic-free, or how much time the animals spent outdoors.

GMO-FREE, NON-GMO, OR NO GMOs

Products can be labeled "GMO-free" if they are produced without being genetically modified through the use of GMOs (genetically modified organisms). Genetic engineering is the process of transferring specific traits or genes from one organism into a different plant or animal.

FARM RAISED FISH

About half of the world's seafood now comes from fish farms, including in the US. Levels of omega-3 fats are reduced by about 50 percent in farmed salmon compared to wild salmon, due to the use of grain and legume feed. Farmed salmon may also spread diseases to wild populations, due to interbreeding with wild species. This threatens the wild gene pool with irreversible bio pollution of contaminants, of which the farmed salmon have high levels. The most commonly farm raised fish besides salmon are tilapia, catfish, "sea" bass and cod.

ORGANIC

In order to be certified organic, the produce must meet the US Department of Agriculture's (USDA) organic standards, and farms and ranches must follow a strict set of guidelines. A third-party certifier inspects these farms and ranches each year to ensure that organic standards are met.

Here are a few of the requirements for organic poultry, cattle and pigs:

- Must be raised organically on certified organic land

- Must be fed certified organic feed

- No antibiotics or added growth hormones are allowed

- Must have outdoor access

- The animals' organic feed cannot contain animal by-products, antibiotics or genetically engineered grains and cannot be grown using persistent pesticides or chemical fertilizers.

Eating organic, Non–GMO, Pasture-raised and cage-free animals is definitely a more expensive option, but the taste is dramatically enhanced, and the boost in nutritional value makes it worthwhile.

These are a few of my favorite main course dishes that are simple and delectable. I strive to use organic, free-range produce as much as possible.

~~~~~~

Grilled Salmon Kebabs

I have adapted this recipe of Natasha Kravchuk, from "Natasha's Kitchen," is quick and easy to prepare. The result is juicy and flavorful salmon that melts in your mouth. You may even want to eat the lemon it's so tasty.

Serves 4

Ingredients
1.5 lbs. salmon fillet, cut into large squares
2 large lemons, thinly sliced
Sixteen 10″ bamboo skewers

Ingredients for the Marinade
2 TB chopped parsley
2 large garlic cloves, minced
½ TB Dijon mustard (I like Grey Poupon)
½ tsp. salt
1/8 tsp ground black pepper
2 TB olive oil, preferably not EVO, as it has a low smoke point
2 TB fresh lemon juice

Directions
Soak the skewers for at least an hour to prevent them from catching fire. Oil the grill then preheat grill to medium, or 375 degrees F.

In a small bowl, stir together all ingredients for the marinade.

Skewer the salmon with the lemon slices folded in half in between each piece of salmon. Use 2 skewers for each kebab as it helps in turning the skewers while cooking.

Place salmon on the grill and grill for 4-5 minutes each side or until cooked through and opaque.

~~~~~~

Herb Crusted Cod
I have made this recipe using a variety of mild white fish such as cod, haddock and lemon sole. The recipe is both simple and delicious, and even non-fish lovers and children seem to enjoy it.

Serves 4

Ingredients
Cod or grouper cut into 6 oz. portions, or 4, 6 oz. pieces haddock
½ cup gluten free panko or quinoa flakes
½ cup fresh chopped herbs such as parsley, dill, basil, chives or tarragon
2 cloves garlic, finely minced

¼ cup olive oil
Salt and pepper to taste

Directions
Preheat oven to 400 degrees F.

Place fillets on a parchment lined baking sheet, and season with salt and pepper. Set aside.

Combine panko, herbs, garlic and olive oil, and spread over the fish.

Place fish in the oven and bake until cooked through, 10 to 12 minutes.

Remove from the oven and serve.

~~~~~~

Roast Lamb and Potatoes with Mint

I have adapted this recipe from Myrna Rosen, and have been making it for years and years. The trick is to use a very good quality olive oil, as well as organic lamb. You will be licking your lips after eating this mouth watering lamb dish.

Ingredients
1 leg of lamb
4-6 cloves garlic, cut in slivers
1 onion cut into slices
2 tsp coarse salt
1 tsp black pepper
2 large sprigs fresh rosemary

¼ cup seeded mustard
½ cup olive oil
½ cup lemon juice
12 pink baby potatoes

Directions

Preheat oven to 400 degrees F.

Wash meat off well. Make incisions all over the meat and insert pieces of garlic and onion deep into the leg.

Mix together all the remaining ingredients and rub well into the lamb, pouring the balance over. Allow to marinade for 24 hours, covered in the refrigerator.

Roast uncovered for 1¾ -2 hours, basting frequently.

Parboil potatoes for 10 minutes, and then place all around the lamb, turning and basting at intervals.

Serve with mint sauce.

Mint Sauce

Chop a few sprigs of mint very finely and mix with ½ cup olive oil, 1 cup brown vinegar, 1 tsp sugar, and a dash of salt and pepper.

Moroccan Chicken with Couscous

This fragrant chicken recipe is adapted from June Edelmuth's book, "Still Hooked on Cooking." I marinade the chicken overnight, or occasionally if possible for two days ahead in the refrigerator, before cooking. The combination of spices and flavors, make this dish particularly exquisite.

The spice mix is usually enough for two separate batches. I usually store the additional spice mix in an airtight container. I substitute the couscous with quinoa for gluten free purposes. Either way, it makes a delightful presentation.

Serves 8-10

Ingredients
1 TB crushed garlic
3 TB cumin
4 tsp. cinnamon
¾ tsp. cayenne pepper
1 TB ground coriander
3 TB paprika
1 ½ tsp. ground cloves
1 TB turmeric
2 TB ground black pepper
1 TB coarse salt
10-12 assorted chicken pieces (I use mostly chicken breast)
1 cup lemon juice
½ cup olive oil

To Serve
1 cup chicken stock
Lemon slices
Fresh coriander sprigs
Jalapeno pepper

Directions
Combine all spice ingredients, except garlic. Crush garlic, rub all over the chicken, and then rub in spice mixture, lemon juice and olive oil and marinade overnight or at least up to 24 hours.

Preheat oven to 350 degrees F, and bake chicken basting every 20 to 30 minutes, until chicken is cooked, about 1 ½ hours.

To serve, heap couscous on a dish and arrange chicken pieces on the sides. Make a gravy by adding 1 cup of chicken stock to the pan, heat through, and pour over the chicken and couscous.

Serve with extra lemon slices, fresh coriander and jalapeno pepper.

Couscous

Ingredients
3 cups couscous (I use Israeli couscous)
1 ½ TB butter
3 tsp.'s chicken stock
3 tsp. lemon rind grated
5 cups boiling water

½ cup pistachio nuts, shelled
½ cup blanched almonds
½ cup raisins

Directions

Just before the chicken is ready, place the couscous, butter, stock powder and grated lemon rind in a bowl. Pour over boiling water, cover and let stand for 5-10 minutes, till all the liquid is absorbed. Fluff with a fork, season to taste with salt and pepper, and mix in nuts and raisins.

Chapter 13

Salad and Vegetables

"Eat food. Not too much. Mostly plants."[16]
- **Michael Pollan**

There are a myriad of different diets available, each one completely different from the next, with more diets being introduced each year. The one thing that most agree on is that vegetables should constitute most of the real estate on your plate. A multitude of delicious vegetables grow throughout the year, the key is to eat them when they are in season and at their freshest, in order to gain their maximum benefit.

We have graduated considerably from the rubbery salads, drowned in dressing, which used to be served as an afterthought at mealtime. Today vegetables are revered for their authentic and unique flavors and textures. Made in a variety of different ways, they provide us with many essential vitamins and minerals. Eating a rainbow of colors every day will also provide us

---

16   Pollan, Michael. *In Defense of Food: Eat Food, Not Too Much, Mostly Plants.* New York: Penguin, 2008. Print.

with important antioxidants, which protect our bodies against free radicals.

When I was on dialysis, I was limited in the vegetables that I could eat. I particularly missed the sweet nutty taste of butternut squash, my favorite winter vegetable. I missed the grounded, satiated feeling I always got after eating it. It also helped with the sweet cravings I developed after my first transplant, once I didn't have to worry about watching my blood sugar anymore.

I also missed eating delicious meaty and juicy tomatoes in the summer. The tomato has been referred to as a "functional food," Food that goes beyond providing just basic nutrition. They aid in preventing chronic disease due to beneficial phytochemicals such as lycopene. Tomatoes are packed full of beneficial nutrients and antioxidants and are a rich source of vitamins A, C and folic acid.

The benefits of consuming fruits and vegetables of all kinds including tomatoes are infinite. As plant food consumption goes up, the risk of heart disease, diabetes, and cancer goes down.

High fruit and vegetable intake is also associated with healthy skin and hair, increased energy and lower weight. It also significantly decreases the risk of obesity and overall mortality.

The following recipes are several of our family favorites.

Roasted Cauliflower, Quinoa and Fennel Salad

This recipe has been adapted from "The Raizons 4" cookbook. Incorporating quinoa into a salad makes it a complete meal because quinoa is a complete protein as well as a carbohydrate. Quinoa is the world's most popular "superfood." It is loaded not only with protein, but with tons of fiber and minerals and doesn't contain any gluten.

I love this recipe as it is not only scrumptious but it keeps and can be eaten a day or two after making it.

Serves 10-12

Ingredients
1 ½ cups water
1 cup quinoa
1 cauliflower, cut in small florets
1 TB sumac
Salt and pepper to taste
Olive oil spray
1 fennel bulb
1 pomegranate, seeded
½ cup currants or raisons
1 cup chopped parsley
½ cup slivered almond, toasted for garnish

Dressing
Juice of 2 lemons
2 TB pomegranate molasses
6 TB olive oil
Salt and pepper

Directions

In a small pot, bring 1 ½ cups water to a boil. Add quinoa, reduce heat, cover and simmer for 10 minutes. Turn off the heat and let stand for another 10 minutes without removing the lid. Place in a large bowl to cool.

Place cauliflower on a baking tray, spray with olive oil, and sprinkle with salt, pepper and sumac. Bake for 40 minutes in 400 degrees F oven for 40 minutes. Set aside to cool.

Pour remaining ingredients in a large bowl with the quinoa.

Whisk dressing ingredients together.

Just before serving, pour dressing over salad and toss gently.

Garnish with toasted almonds.

~~~~~~~~~~~~~~~~~~~~~~~~~~~~~~~~~~~~~

Maple Roasted Butternut Squash and Apple Salad

We love making this salad in the fall, particularly for Thanksgiving. Pure maple syrup is the healthiest type of sweetener you can use. It has been consumed for many centuries in North America, since the times of the Native Americans.

Serves 8

Ingredients
1 small butternut squash, peeled and cut into 2 ½ inch chunks
3 Granny Smith apples, cored and chopped
1-2 TB olive oil
1 TB pure maple syrup
1 tsp. kosher salt
½ tsp. course ground black pepper
¼ cup dried cranberries
Mixed baby lettuce, about 8-10 cups
½ cup pepitas
¾ cup feta sheep's milk feta cheese

Maple dressing
2 cloves garlic
1 TB Dijon mustard
1 TB brown grainy mustard
1/2 cup pure maple syrup
1/3 cup apple cider vinegar
1 cup olive oil
1 shallot
Salt and pepper to taste

Directions
Preheat oven to 425 degrees F.

Place the apple and butternut squash in a roasting pan, mix well with the maple syrup, salt and pepper, and roast for 30-40 minutes, till easily pierced with a fork. Allow to cool. Mix all other ingredients.

Combine dressing ingredients and use an immersion blender to blend until smooth.

Pour dressing over the salad, and serve.

～～～～～～～～～～～～～～～～

Simple Israeli Salad

This simple, delicious salad is a staple in every Israeli home, at every meal. It is refreshing and substantial at the same time. The acidity of the lemon juice combined with the sweetness and umami of the tomatoes, and the richness of the olive oil, make this salad a wonderful accompaniment to every meal.

Serves 4-6

Ingredients
3 cups chopped tomatoes
3 cups chopped mini cucumbers
1 small red onion chopped
¼ cup chopped parsley
2 TB olive oil
2 tsp lemon juice
2 tsp white balsamic vinegar
1 tsp coarse salt
Pepper to taste

Directions
Place all ingredients in a bowl, toss well and serve immediately.

Rainbow Detox Salad

This has become a staple in our household ever since I made this recipe for a cooking class I gave several years ago. The seeds are packed with protein and make this into a complete satisfying meal, along with the combination of ingredients and textures.

Ingredients

3 carrots, peeled and shredded
1 beetroot, peeled and shredded
1 bunch kale, hard rib removed and shredded
1 packet brussel sprouts, shaved
6 scallions, cut on the diagonal
1-2 avocado, cubed
2 TB pumpkin seeds
2 TB sunflower seeds
1 TB sesame seeds

Dressing

2 TB honey
2 TB apple cider vinegar
1 tsp sesame oil
1 TB fresh ginger
Juice of 1 lemon or lime
1-2 TB soy sauce or liquid Amino's (gluten free soy option)
1 tsp salt

Directions

Mix all salad ingredients together except seeds.

Whisk dressing ingredients together and pour over salad about half an hour before serving.

Add seeds and adjust seasonings just before serving

~~~~~~

Wilted Kale with Garlic and Mushrooms

This is simple, quick and delicious. No more needs to be said!

Serves 4

Ingredients
2 TB olive oil
8 oz. shiitake mushrooms, stems removed and thinly sliced
2 cloves garlic, minced
1 large bunch dinosaur kale, cleaned, rib removed and chopped. You can substitute with other greens, such as spinach or Swiss chard.

Directions
In a small sauté pan, heat 1 TB olive oil over medium heat. Add mushrooms and cook until softened, 6-8 minutes. Add garlic and cook another 2 minutes. Remove from pan and set aside. Add remaining 1 TB olive oil to the pan and heat over medium heat, add kale and toss, cooking about 5 minutes. Add shiitake/garlic mix and reheat. Add salt and pepper to taste.

Roasted Brussel Sprouts, with Fennel and Shiitake Mushrooms

Adapted from Terry Walters, "Eat Clean, Live Well".
Brussels sprouts change in density and flavor after roasting. They become more dense, soft and delicious, particularly when combined with the other caramelized vegetables. Brussels sprouts are a rich source of antioxidants. They are rich in antiviral and antibiotic properties.

Serves 6

Ingredients
1 ½ pounds brussels sprouts, trimmed and cut in half
4 shallots, peeled and thinly sliced
½ pound shiitake mushroom caps, wiped clean, stem removed
1 large fennel bulb, trim, washed and thinly sliced
5 garlic cloves, peeled
¼ cup extra virgin olive oil
3 TB balsamic vinegar
2 TB fresh rosemary

Directions
Preheat oven to 425 degrees F.

Place all vegetables in a large baking tray. Toss with olive oil, balsamic vinegar, rosemary, and add coarse salt and pepper to taste.

Place in the oven and roast for 25 minutes. Stir and roast for a further 20-25 minutes. Adjust seasonings and serve.

Chapter 15

Nutritious Smoothies

A smoothie for breakfast, post workout, or as a mid-afternoon snack to tide you over until dinner, is an effortless, and energizing way of ensuring that you get adequate greens and fiber into your diet. Eating greens in the morning is a wonderful way of alkalizing and detoxifying your body, as well as reducing inflammation.

Cruciferous vegetables, such as kale, watercress and arugula—just to name a few, are abundant in carotenoids and are powerful antioxidants. They also have an unusually high content of Vitamin C, Vitamin A and manganese. When eaten fresh and raw, as in salads or smoothies, nutrients from the cruciferous vegetables are more likely to be absorbed in the upper digestive tract, transported to the liver, and made available to other tissues in the body that might benefit from them. Berries are high in nutritional value, while remaining low in calories, and are perfect for smoothie making. They have the highest antioxidant capacity of all commonly consumed fruits and vegetables. The flavonoids present in blueberries, are major antioxidant compounds. They protect against DNA damage, which is a leading driver of aging and cancer. The antioxidants in blueberries also help improve brain function.

Smoothies are delicious, filling and hydrating. Add a scoop of nut butter, coconut oil or avocado for a healthy fat or a nut milk for a superb source of protein, and a small amount of fruit for sweetness.

They are an excellent means of blood sugar control when using the correct combination of protein, fat and carbohydrates. The fiber content not only improves digestion and blood sugar, but also begins the digestive process by "chewing" your food for you, allowing your digestive system to rest.

Yes, eating healthy and tasting great can go hand in hand. These three recipes are my favorite palate pleasing ones. You can also make up your own recipes, choosing your favorite ingredients.

~~~~~~~~~~~~~~~~

Mint Chocolate Chip Smoothie
This detoxifying smoothie is healthy, nutritious and tastes like dessert.

Serves 1

Ingredients
1 to 2 scoops chocolate protein powder (I use Dr. Axe's brand)
1 cup unsweetened coconut or almond milk
½ cup fresh mint leaves
4/5 ice cubes

½ cup spinach or kale (I steam my kale slightly to reduce bitterness)
¼ cup fresh cocoa nibs
1 TB coconut oil or avocado

Directions

Blend all ingredients in a Vitamix or high powered blender. Consistency should be creamy and thick. Eat immediately, or store in the refrigerator for later in the day. Garnish with finely chopped mint leaves.

Anti-Aging Berry Smoothie

This recipe is loaded with antioxidants and healthy fats. It is a perfect breakfast or post workout snack.

Serves 1

Ingredients

½ banana
1 cup mixed berries (fresh or frozen)
½ cup unsweetened almond or coconut milk
1 TB fresh ground flax seeds
1 TB raw almond butter
4 ice cubes

Directions

Combine all ingredients except flax seeds in a Vitamix, and blend. Add flax seeds last. You may need to add additional berries if the mixture is too thin. Consistency should be smooth and thick.

Green Apple Smoothie

This tart and healing smoothie, makes a delicious breakfast.

Serves 1-2

Ingredients

1 cup kale, raw or lightly steamed to avoid bitterness
1 cup spinach
1 green apple cored
1/2 cucumber
½ lemon (squeezed)
½ bananas
5 ice cubes
1 TB fresh ground flax seeds
1 tsp fresh ginger (grated)

Blend in a Vitamix and serve.

Chapter 16

Gluten-Free Baking

Humans have been eating wheat, and therefore gluten, for at least decades. For people with celiac disease, about one percent of the population, exposure to gluten can trigger an immune reaction powerful enough to severely damage the villi, or brush like surfaces of the small intestine.

But there are many people suffering with various forms of autoimmunity that have non-celiac gluten sensitivity. Celiac disease often affects people with irritable bowel syndrome (IBS), neuropathy (nerve pains or numbness), autoimmune disease (RA, MS, Crohn's, type 1 diabetes, etc.) and inflammation, such as Lyme and fibromyalgia. Side effects may include bloating, gas, brain fog, rashes, eczema and leaky gut syndrome to name a few. David Perlmutter, a neurologist and author of the gluten-free movement's foundational texts, "Grain Brain: The Surprising Truth About Wheat, Carbs, and Sugar—Your Brain's Silent Killers," explains this and more in his book. Gluten sensitivity, he writes, "Represents one of the greatest and most under-recognized health threats to humanity." Around twenty million people, or six to 10 percent of people in the U.S., complain that they regularly experience distress after eating products containing gluten, while a third of American adults are trying to eliminate it from their diets.[17]

Cutting out gluten from your diet may seem like a daunting and limiting task. Fortunately, there are many healthy and delicious foods that are naturally gluten-free. In fact, the most cost-effective and healthiest way to follow a gluten-free diet is to seek out naturally gluten-free food groups, such as fruits, vegetables, beans, legumes, nuts, and protein sources, such as meat, poultry and fish, as well as some dairy.

Gluten-free foods are usually not enriched and are often higher in sugar and starches. Gluten is found in grains, such as wheat, barley, rye and a combination of wheat and rye called triticale.

There are many naturally gluten-free grains that you can enjoy in a variety of creative ways. Many of these grains can be easily found in local grocery stores, but some of the lesser-known grains may only be found at specialty or health food stores. I do not recommend purchasing grains from bulk bins because of possible cross-contamination with gluten.

The following are gluten-free substitutes for traditional grains and flour.

- rice
- cassava

- corn
- potato

---

17   Perlmutter, David. *Grain Brain.* N.p.: n.p., n.d. Web.

- tapioca
- beans
- sorghum
- quinoa
- millet
- buckwheat groats (also known as kasha)
- soy
- arrowroot
- amaranth
- teff
- flax
- chia
- yucca
- gluten-free oats
- nut flours

Many products that usually contain gluten now have gluten-free alternatives available in most grocery stores, which make living gluten-free much easier. Proper "gluten-free" labeling is important. It is also important to remember that "wheat-free" or sprouted wheat, does not mean "gluten-free." Always check labels to make sure that the ingredients are pronounceable, and not full of sugar, starches or chemicals. Barley can be found on a label in the form of malt, malt flavoring, beer or brewer's yeast.

Gluten-free bread can often be found in the freezer section. There are also gluten-free flours and flour blends available, allowing you to bake your own bread. I am including a few gluten free recipes that I love, and make frequently.

Gluten-Free Banana Bread with Chocolate Chips

This recipe from the gluten-free goddess, Karina Allich, is absolutely delicious. I encourage one-and-all to check out her gluten-free recipes, they are fabulous! This is by far the best gluten-free banana and chocolate chip recipe around, and I have tried many of them. This recipe is not only gluten free, it is dairy free, egg free, soy free and nut free, and if using vegan chocolate chips, is a vegan recipe too. I always feel guilty throwing out over ripe bananas, so I pop them in the freezer until I am ready to use them. Steve is a chocolate cake lover and he loves this recipe.

Serves 8

Ingredients
3 ripe bananas
1/3 cup coconut oil
¾ cup organic brown sugar or pure maple syrup
2 tsp vanilla extract
1 ½ cups gluten free flour, or gluten free baking mix
¼ cup flax seed
1 tsp baking soda, heaped
2 ½ tsp. baking powder, heaped
Pinch of salt
½ tsp. xanthan gum
1 heaped tsp cinnamon
½ cup dark or semi-sweet chocolate chips

Directions

Preheat oven to 350 degrees F.

Combine wet ingredients in a food processor. Add the dry ingredients, and mix till smooth. If the batter looks too thin, add more gluten-free flour, a tablespoon at a time, till thicker. Place in a mixing bowl.

Add chocolate chips by hand and stir to blend

Lightly oil a standard loaf pan and dust with corn flour. Pour batter into the loaf pan and place in the center of the preheated oven for an hour, or till it is crusty and firm and a wooden pick inserted into the middle emerges clean.

Cool on a wire rack. Slice when cool. This freezes well.

~~~~~~~~~~~~~~~~~~~~~~~~~~~~~~~~~~~

Fabulous Superfood Banana Health Bread

This delicious recipe is from "One Green Planet" by Margaret Mouton. It is also vegan as well as gluten-free, and is packed with oats, chia seeds, sunflower seeds and other ingredients that are so healthy for you. This bread is also packed with fiber that is great for digestion. It is thoroughly delicious.

Serves 8-10

Ingredients
4 large or 5 small bananas
1 ½ cup non-dairy milk
1 ½ cups gluten-free oats
1 ¼ cup oat or brown rice flour
1/3 cup honey or pure maple syrup
4 TB coconut oil
2 tsp baking powder
2 tsp baking soda
2 TB chia seeds
1 TB flax seeds
1/3 cup mix of dried cranberries, sunflower seeds and pepitas, plus an extra ¼ cup for the topping

Directions
Preheat the oven to 350 degrees F.

Place all dry ingredients in a bowl and mix well.

In a food processor, blend bananas with coconut oil and honey, then add the milk.

Add dry ingredients to the mixture and blend well and place in a mixing bowl.

Lastly add dried cranberries, sunflower seeds and pepitas and blend.

Place in the loaf pan that has been lightly oiled and dusted with corn flour.

Press the topping gently with the palm of your hand onto the top of the loaf.

Place in the center of the oven and bake for 30 minutes. Allow to cool completely before slicing.

This can be sliced and stored in the freezer.

~~~~~~

Pear, Cranberry Ginger Crumble

I have adapted this recipe by Deb Perelman from "Smitten Kitchen" to be gluten free. It is simply delectable!

Serves 10-12

Ingredients

Crumble

1 cup gluten-free flour
¼ cup granulated sugar
3 TB dark or light brown sugar
1 cup gluten-free ginger cookies (store bought), crumbled
1/8 tsp ground ginger
1/8 tsp table salt
Pinch of white pepper, particularly if you don't like your ginger cookies too spicy
½ cup unsalted butter

Filling

1 pound, or about 4/5 large ripe pears, peeled, cored and sliced ¼ inch thick – I use whichever type pear looks firm and fresh, usually Anjou or Bosc
1 ½ cups fresh or frozen cranberries
1 TB lemon juice

½ tsp finely grated lemon zest
½ tsp vanilla essence (make sure it is gluten free)
½ cup granulated sugar
2 TB cornstarch

Directions
Preheat the oven to 350 degrees F.

Stir together the flour, granulated sugar, brown sugar, ginger cookie crumbles, ginger, salt and pepper. Stir in melted butter until large crumbs form.

In a 1 ½ to 2 quart baking dish, mix the pears, cranberries, lemon juice and zest, and vanilla. In a small bowl whisk the sugar and cornstarch together, then toss with the fruit mixture in the baking dish.

Sprinkle the ginger mixture on top of the fruit. Set the dish on a foil lined baking sheet, and bake for 45 minutes until the crumble is browned and bubbling through the crumbs. Serve warm.

I like to serve this with a scoop of coconut sorbet.

~~~~~~~~~~~~~~~~~~~~~~~~~~~~~~~~~~~~~~

Great, Simple Flourless Chocolate Cake

This recipe from "The Raizons Four" cookbook, is another favorite. It is simple, quick and delicious. It is great for Passover, as well as gluten-free baking.

Serves 8-10

Ingredients

7 oz. Bittersweet or semi-sweet chocolate chips, chopped (I use a good quality chocolate, which enhances the flavor.)

¾ cup powdered sugar

1 tsp. coffee powder

¾ cup sticks unsalted butter

6 large eggs, separated

2 ¼ cups almond flour

Coconut oil spray

Extra powdered sugar for dusting

Directions

Preheat oven to 325 degrees F.

Place chocolate, sugar, butter and coffee powder into a heatproof bowl. Place over a pot of simmering water. Stir regularly until the chocolate and the butter have melted. Remove from the heat and set aside to cool for 5 minutes.

In a separate bowl, beat egg whites until stiff.

Place chocolate mixture into the mixing bowl of a Mixmaster or food processor. Add egg yolks and mix well. Add almond meal and mix until well combined. Add a few spoons of egg whites to the chocolate mixture. With the machine on low speed, gently fold to loosen the mixture. Remove bowl from the machine and gently fold in remaining egg whites by hand.

Line a spring form tin (12 inch) with baking paper and spray sides with coconut oil spray. Pour mixture into the tin and bake for 40-50 minutes, or until a skewer emerges clean from the middle. Dust with powdered sugar.

Can be served with raspberry sauce or coconut ice cream, or just on its own.

Chapter 17

Sweet Endings

Having been raised In South Africa, I am accustomed to afternoon tea, served at 4PM daily. There would be an array of cakes, cookies and something savory, for those, like me, who were not supposed to eat sweets, set out on the table. Although savory food is satisfying in a deep, soulful way, the allure of dessert is an intoxicating slice of heaven, and almost impossible to resist.

I would be remiss if I did not mention my mother regarding dessert and sweets. Mom has always been a compulsive sugar eater. She would set aside time each week to bake several batches of cookies to serve to guests for tea. One of my earliest childhood kitchen memories, is of helping her roll out the dough, every surface in the kitchen covered in flour, to cut out shapes for cookies.

My mother was a wonderful cook, but baking was her specialty. She would glimpse at a recipe, and then throw in ingredients of her own choosing, estimating quantities, and always allowing for her own improvisation.

Magically, her creations always seemed to turn out brilliantly. Wherever she went, whether she was going to a doctor's office, her beautician, or simply to visit with a friend, she always took a tray of her delicious muffins that were hard to resist.

Now that I am able to enjoy desserts, I try to keep the sugar intake on the desserts I make low, as well as the other ingredients that are not particularly kind to us. Most of my recipes are therefore full of healthy ingredients, but still taste decadent.

These are a few of my favorites:

~~~~~~

No Bake Cookies

Is there such a thing as a healthy cookie? This is my idea of a cookie that not only tastes delicious, but is super healthy too. Whenever I make these, they are gone in a few hours, they are just so good.

Serves 8

Ingredients
¼ cup unsalted butter
½ cup almond butter or tahini
¼ cup almond milk
½ cup maple syrup or honey
1 ½ cups gluten free cooking oats
2 TB golden flaxseed
½ cup bittersweet chocolate chips

Directions

In a medium saucepan combine butter, almond butter or tahini, milk and syrup and cook over medium heat stirring constantly. Remove from the heat once the butter is melted and allow to cool.

Stir in the oats and the flaxseed.

Once the mixture has cooled slightly, stir in the chocolate chips. Drop spoonful size quantities onto parchment-lined cookie trays and leave for an hour to harden.

~~~~~~

Tiramisu

This dessert from Levana Kirschenbaum's book "Levana's Table", is just fabulous. Don't tell anyone that it is made with tofu, let them taste it first. I recommend using organic tofu, as soybeans are the most commonly genetically modified crops. It is shockingly delicious, and healthy as well. Is there really such a thing as a healthy dessert? Try it out for yourself and see.

It is best to use sponge cake rather than lady fingers because it maintains its shape better when soaked in the espresso and brandy. Lining the mold with plastic wrap allows very easy unmolding, just pull up the sides, and the cake lifts right out. Use the best quality chocolate if possible. This dessert is best made a few hours before or even the day before, to give it time to soak up all the flavors.

Serves 12

Ingredients
1 ¼ pounds store bought sponge cake
1 pound silken organic tofu, thoroughly drained and dried with layers of paper towel
2 TB oil
½ cup sugar
1 container Tofutti cream cheese
2½ TB espresso or coffee powder, dissolved in 2/3 cup hot water
¼ cup brandy, rum or bourbon
8 oz. best quality semi-sweet chocolate, chopped

Directions
Preheat oven to 375 degrees F.

Slice the cake in half inch thick pieces and toast in the oven for about 15 minutes, turning the slices over once, until medium brown on all sides. Let cool.

In a food processor, process the tofu with the oil and sugar and process until smooth. Add the cream cheese. Pour mixture into a bowl.

Combine the coffee mixture and the brandy in a container with a spout, like a glass measuring cup.

Grease a 2 quart (8 cup) loaf pan and line with plastic wrap, letting the sides overhang. Line the bottom completely with slices of cake, trimmed to fit tightly. Pour half the coffee mixture evenly and carefully over the cake.

Spread half of the tofu mixture evenly over the cake, and sprinkle with half the grated chocolate over the tofu mixture. Repeat: cake, coffee, tofu mixture and chocolate.

Fold overhanging plastic wrap towards the center of the mold.

Refrigerate for a few hours until set. Unmold and slice.

~~~~~~~~~~~~~~~~~~~~~~~~

Persian Chocolate Bark with Cardamom and Coffee

This sensational recipe makes a perfect hostess gift. The recipe is courtesy of Laura Zinn Fromm's book "Sweet Survival" and has become my all-time favorite chocolate recipe. The key is to use very good quality chocolate. It is super easy and takes all of 15 minutes to prepare. Mulberries are small, soft shriveled fruit, much like blueberries, and are available online or at specialty grocery stores. I have substituted dried blueberries, and they taste great too. There is no added sugar in the recipe, which makes it a perfect choice to satisfy that chocolate craving. Be warned though, this is an addictive recipe.

Serves 8-10

Ingredients
2 cups semi-sweet chocolate chips, I use unsweetened dark chocolate
1 tsp ground cardamom

¼ cup dried mulberries
¼ cup dried tart cherries, I sometimes use ½ cup if I
have them available
¾ cup almonds, toasted and coarsely chopped
½ cup pistachios, toasted and coarsely chopped
2 tsp coffee beans, coarsely chopped
Pinch of coarse salt, preferably sea salt

Directions

Grease a baking sheet and line with parchment paper

Melt chocolate in a saucepan over simmering water. Add cardamom and stir to dissolve for a few minutes. Turn off the heat and stir in half the mulberries, cherries, almonds and pistachios.

Pour chocolate onto prepared baking sheet. With a spatula, spread chocolate in a wide rectangle and ¼ inch thick. Sprinkle with the remaining nuts, dried fruit and ground coffee beans, and press into the chocolate. Dust with salt.

Cool in the refrigerator for about 2 hours, until hard. When firm, slide chocolate onto a cutting board and break into pieces. The chocolate gets soft quickly so keep refrigerated until just before serving.

Conclusion

"Tragedy should be utilized as a source of strength.
No matter what sort of difficulties,
how painful experience is, if we lose our hope,
that's our real disaster." [18]
Dalai Lama XIV

Whether you are struggling to maintain balance dealing with a chronic disease like type 1 diabetes, or you are on dialysis, and waiting for a transplant, my message remains consistent. Even on the darkest of days, never give up hope and continue pursuing your dreams.

Make an all-out effort to not allow fear to paralyze you into being powerless. We all have strength beyond measure, even under the worst of circumstances. Keep moving forward, and do the best that you can to manage your disease.

Don't forget that you are never alone. If you do not have the luxury of family close by, there are online communities, and support groups, that can relate to what you are dealing with, and offer support. There is no humiliation in reaching out for help to a professional

18   Dalai Lama XIVI "Continued Hope." *Continued Hope.* N.p., n.d. Web. 11 Mar. 2016.

with expertise in dealing with your condition, such as a psychologist, or a health coach. Part of healing and maintaining good health is having a good attitude and a healthy mind. Getting support helps you to acknowledge what it is you are struggling with, and move forward with determination.

Accept that being a type 1 diabetic is not your fault. There is no room for embarrassment or guilt. Yes complications are always a possibility, but it is also possible to lead a full, happy and healthy life, despite the complications.

For years I felt embarrassed to reveal my left arm, which bears the evidence of a dialysis graft. It would be 100 degrees outside, and my arms would still be covered. I have finally begun to wear my scars with pride, as my badge of honor. It is remarkable just how liberating it is to finally let go of the shame.

Make sure that you nourish your body, with both primary and secondary food. Primary food is what nourishes us on an emotional level, and secondary food is the food that we eat. It is within your power to control the food on your plate, as well as what nourishes you on a much deeper, spiritual level. The tools that are available to make living with diabetes easier are so much more sophisticated than they were when I was diagnosed. All you need is the motivation to utilize these tools and to take control.

Living with type 1 diabetes is not about being perfect all the time. There are going to be occasional hills and valleys, no matter what you do. Diabetes can be unpredictable at times. But the important thing to remember is to be kind to yourself, and to keep moving forward without allowing diabetes to define who you are at your core.

Although living with type 1 diabetes and the associated complications takes consistent hard work, there is always room for joy, growth and compassion within both yourself and your loved ones.

For those who are healthy, I cannot stress enough the importance of becoming an organ donor. It has saved mine as well as countless other lives worldwide. Signing up on your state registry means that someday you too could save lives as a donor—by leaving behind the gift of life. When you register, most states let you choose what organs and tissues you want to donate, and you can update your status at any time.

You can sign up online at organdonor.gov or in-person at your local motor vehicle department. Registering online takes just a few minutes of your time, and can change the quality of someone's life for a lifetime.

Acknowledgements

Thank you to my loving husband, for encouraging me through the process of writing this book. Steve lovingly helped me edit the book and listened patiently to all the rewrites. I am so grateful to have such a loving, supportive husband, who advocated for me when I couldn't. It is because of him that I am alive today.

Thank you to my daughter, Gaby, for being the inspiration and motivation behind everything I do. You are the light in my life.

Thank you to my sister, Bonita, for always encouraging and believing in me. Her love and support has been unending. I also give thanks to my niece, Leigh for helping me with editing. Your contribution has been invaluable and I am truly grateful.

I give particular thanks to my mother, for lovingly taking care of me as a child, the best way she could. Her trips to bring me school lunches every day, and her unconditional care and love, even when she was scared, have not gone unappreciated. I am deeply grateful to her, for inspiring me in cooking.

Our sincerest gratitude to Edward and Rose Dreyer, as well as to the late Anne Dreyer, for their unwavering love and support since our arrival in the USA. We are truly grateful to all our family and friends around the world, especially to my brother Steve and sister-in-law Pearl, who came to our support at a critical time. Particular thanks go to my dear friend Debbie Russ, as well as to Marie Becker and Barbara Rubin for being our surrogate family when we needed it the most.

A huge shout out goes to Belinda Ossip and to the Institute for Integrative Nutrition for awakening my passion and inspiring me to grow and develop beyond my imagination. I also appreciate the "Launch your Dream Book," course and Lyndsey Smith for inspiring me to take time and write this book. It has made my dream a reality. I could not have done it without you.

Thank you also to Levana Kirschenbaum, June Edelmuth, Sharon Glass, the Raizon sisters in Melbourne, Laura Zinn Fromm and all the other contributors to the recipes listed in this book. Your superb recipes are a continual inspiration to me. They nourish me on every level.

I give a lot of thanks to all my doctors at The University of Minnesota Hospital, Emory University Hospital, Johns Hopkins Hospital and Mount Sinai Hospital for taking such amazing care of me. Antonio Guasch. MD from Emory Hospital deserves special mention, as does Andy Drexler, MD. Their commitment and kindness do not go unappreciated. I have been able to accomplish everything because of all of you.

Lastly, I give thanks to my transplanted kidney and pancreas. They have proved to me that there is life post-transplant.

Transplanted

Recipe Index

SOUP

SALADS

VEGETABLES

GLUTEN-FREE BAKING

DESSERTS

NUTRITIOUS SMOOTHIES

Resources and Works Cited

"The Autoimmune Solution: Prevent and Reverse the Full Spectrum of Inflammatory Symptoms and Diseases by Amy Myers." *Free Book® PDF Books Library to Download EBooks*. N.p., n.d. Web. 13 Mar. 2016.

"Continued Hope." *Continued Hope*. N.p., n.d. Web. 11 Mar. 2016.

Diabetes Summit. Prod. Brian Mowll. Perf. Kerri Spaarling. N.p., Web. 30 Mar. 2015.

Edelmuth, June. " *Hooked on Cooking"by June Edelmuth*. N.p., 2000. Web. 14 Mar. 2016.

"The Effect of Intensive Treatment of Diabetes on the Development and Progression of Long-Term Complications in Insulin-Dependent Diabetes Mellitus — NEJM." *New England Journal of Medicine*. N.p., n.d. Web. 13 Mar. 2016.

National Eye Institute, Facts about Diabetic Eye Disease: Sept, 2015: http//nei.nih.gov/health/diabetic/retinopathy.

"Food & Wine Recipes | MyRecipes.com." *MyRecipes. com.* N.p., n.d. Web. 14 Mar. 2016.

Fromm, Laura Zinn. *Sweet Survival: Tales of Cooking & Coping.* N.p.: n.p., n.d. Print.

Glass, Sharon. "Simply Delicious." *Alibris.* N.p., 2000. Web. 14 Mar. 2016.

Glass, Sharon. "Simply Too Delicious" – 31 Dec 2002. N.p., 2002. Web. 14 Mar. 2016.

Glass, Sharon. "Absolutely Delicious"—2005.N.p.Web. 15Mar.2016

"Grain Brain Describes the Staggering Effects of Carbs on the Brain." *David Perlmutter MD.* N.p.,

"The Institute for Integrative Nutrition." *Institute for Integrative Nutrition.* N.p., n.d. Web. 13

Kirschenmbaum, Levana. "Robot Check." *Robot Check.* N.p., 2002. Web. 14 Mar. 2016.

"Long Walk To Freedom: The Autobiography of Nelson Mandela Paperback – 12 Oct 1995.".

Lorenzo Benet, The Kidney Cha. People Magazine Article Nov 30, 2009, pg70 "People Magaine."

"Making Healthy Food Choices." *American Diabetes Association.* N.p., n.d. Web. 13 Mar. 2016.

Mayo clinic staff, , diabetes-symptoms, http://www. mayoclinic.org/diseases-conditions/diabetes/ indepth/June 2013

NKF, 2015 https://www.kidney.org/about/contact Paltrow, Gwyneth. *My Fathers Daughter*. N.p.: n.p., 2011. Print.

Perelman, Deb. *Smitten Kitchen RSS*. N.p., n.d. Web. 14 Mar. 2016.

Pollan, Michael. *Cooked, A Natural History of Transformation*. London: Allen Lane, 2013. Print.

Pollan, Michael. *Food Rules: An Eater's Manual*. New York: Penguin, 2009. Print.

Pollan, Michael. *In Defense of Food: Eat Food, Not Too Much, Mostly Plants*. New York: Penguin, 2008. Print.

Raizon,"Raizons 4," Lana and Delia. N.p., 2013. Web. "Recipes – "NatashasKitchen.com." N.p., n.d. Web. 14 Mar. 2016.

"http://www.sciencedirect.com/science/.com" *Elsevier: Article Locator*. D Stress as a Trigger for Autoimmunity, n.d. Web. 13 Mar. 2016.

"Sodium and Your CKD Diet: How to Spice Up Your Cooking." *The National Kidney Foundation*. N.p., 07 Jan. 2016. Web. 13 Mar. 2016.

Steel Magnolias. Dir. Herbert Ross. Perf. Sally Field, Dolly Parton, Julia Roberts, Daryl Hannah, Olympia Dukakis, Shirley MacLaine, Tom Skerritt, and Sam Shepard. Tri-Star, 1989.

"Waiting, Pre-Transplant." *The National Kidney Foundation*. N.p., 12 Aug. 2014. Web. 13 Mar. 2016.

Walters, Terry. "Terry Walters Eat Clean Live Well." *Terry Walters*. N.p., n.d. Web. 14 Mar. 2016.

This book was inspired by my experience at the *Institute for Integrative Nutrition*® (IIN) where I received my training in holistic wellness and health coaching. IIN offers a truly comprehensive **Health Coach Training Program** that invites students to deeply explore the things that are most nourishing to them. From the physical aspects of nutrition and eating wholesome foods that work best for each individual person, to the concept of Primary Food – the idea that everything in life including our spirituality, career, relationships, and fitness contribute to our inner and outer health.

IIN helped me reach optimal health and balance. This inner journey unleashed the passion that compelled me to share what I've learnt and inspire others to take control of their health, by implementing my "balance your blood sugar" program.

From renowned wellness experts as Visiting Teachers to the convenience of their online learning platform, this school has changed my life and I believe it will do the same for you. I invite you to learn more about the **Institute for Integrative Nutrition** and explore how the Health Coach Training Program can help you transform your life.

Feel free to contact me to learn more about my personal experience at www.janicezundehealth.com. The website also includes information about my services, programs, upcoming events and cooking classes.

About Janice

Janice Zunde is a Certified Holistic Health Coach, passionate cook, wife, mother and author. Janice has always gravitated towards healing professions, with a background in science, and studied Orthoptics at the University of the Witwatersrand Medical School, in South Africa. She did her training at 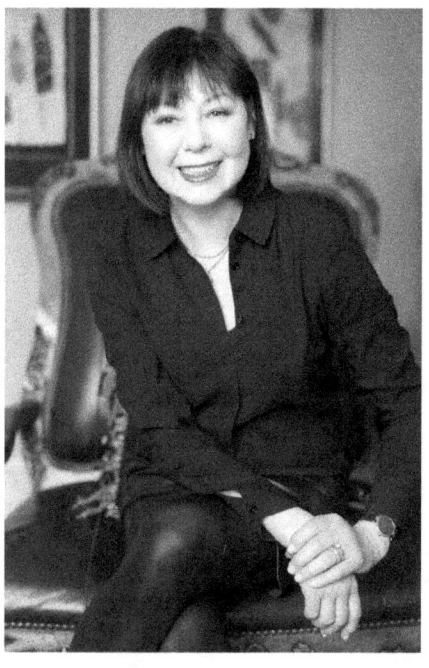 the Institute of Integrative Nutrition®, in NYC. Janice has expertise in dealing with the challenges of type 1 diabetes and kidney failure. For more information on Janice or to stay in the know of her upcoming events check out her website, www.janicezundehealth.com, or email her at janzundehealth@gmail.com. The book is available on Amazon or you can buy the book on Janice's website.